Dr. Paul Saba is a Canadian colleague in search of the meaning of medicine, the meaning of life, and the nonsense of death. He stumbles against a society where selfishness has become the only accepted value under the banner of the right to individual self-determination.

After the legalization of the right to forbid a baby's preborn right to life, it was to be expected that the policy would extend to the elimination of a person after birth. Although some doctors are complying with these laws, this is contrary to their code of medical ethics.

In this context of physician collaborators who are acting against humanity, the work of Dr. Paul Saba shows tremendous courage, tenacity, and exceptional humanity.

—Georges Casteur, M.D.
Former Medical Superintendent, BZIO
(Rehabilitation Hospital, Ostend, Belgium)
Past Chairman, Medical Board of West Flanders

I was honoured to interview Dr. Paul Saba for *Katolskt magasin*—the only Catholic news magazine in Sweden—recently, and I have since had the opportunity to read his new book, *Made to Live*. The book is an engaging and very personal story about the reason for Dr. Saba's conviction that every country or jurisdiction that legalizes Medical Aid in Dying (MAiD) is making a fatal mistake.

Dr. Saba's extensive experience as a doctor—as well as his third child being born with a very serious heart condition—has formed his conviction that allowing doctors to kill patients at their request is always gravely wrong. He has followed this conviction and has fought a number of legal battles in Canada against euthanasia, both before and after the legalization of MAiD. He speaks with a rare, personal conviction that is never boring to the reader, and manages to balance factual and personal arguments.

I fully recommend this book to everyone—especially all those who think that the issue of Medical Aid in Dying does not have very much to do with their lives. They may be faced with this issue sooner than they think.

—Helena D'Arcy
Author, Sweden

Dr. Paul Saba's personal journey to save life demonstrates his caring heart not only for his family but all those around him in the world whom he considers part of his extended family. He recognizes assisted suicide and euthanasia are neither caring nor compassionate.

—Nancy Elliott
Euthanasia Prevention Coalition USA

In this book, we see Dr. Paul Saba as a loving father, a practicing physician and a devout believer in life. He presents facts and arguments, but also personal experiences which show why a civilized society should never open the door to euthanasia.

—Per Ewert
Director, Clapham Institute, Sweden

Dr. Paul Saba's journey for life should inspire everyone who reads his book and cause those who may be considering abortion, assisted suicide, or euthanasia to pause and reevaluate their decision. My personal experience has taught me that some of our decisions are life-changing and cannot be reversed. Dr. Paul Saba combines his professional insights with personal experience to shape a deep, principled defense of the most vulnerable members of our communities, each one unique and precious. This is a book that will impact me for years to come.

—Catherine Glenn Foster, M.A., J.D.
President & CEO, Americans United for Life

The book you are about to read could be considered one of the most significant literary works of our time addressing the issue of euthanasia and assisted suicide. This issue is plaguing our nation's collective mindset, which sadly is determined to model for the world a progressive culture. In *Made to Live*, Dr. Paul Saba has articulated with clarity an academic, intellectual, moral, and spiritual argument promoting life and living with dignity, providing end of life care that honours life and the natural process of dying. From his wealth of wisdom and life experiences as a medical physician, he exposes the erroneous and diabolical strategies that promote ending life as a convenient solution by debunking the five myths that govern and legitimize assisted suicide by medical practitioners and patients. His response to them is brilliant, leaving no doubt in the mind of any reader that there is never any justification for euthanasia or assisted suicide.

Thank you, Dr. Saba, for your excellent work in writing with wisdom, compassion, and sensitivity. Well done.

—Rev. Giulio Lorefice Gabeli
Senior Pastor, Westwood Church, Vancouver, B.C.

Dr. Paul Saba's book, *Made to Live*, beats heroically against the powerful currents of fatalism and materialism that dominate our culture. These inspirational pages are filled with wisdom and boundless humanity, as he illuminates the true nature of compassion and dignity in treating society's most vulnerable members. We should all be so lucky to have our own version of Dr. Saba at our side—and on our side—during the loneliest stage of life's journey.

—Barbara Kay
Journalist & Author, Canada

It has been my privilege to get to know Dr. Paul Saba, both as my doctor and a frequent guest in the German-English congregation I served as Senior Pastor.

The congregation of Full Gospel Assembly Lachine has been encouraged and moved by his passion for life and truth, as well as by the oath he took to do no harm.

I was impressed with his presentation before the court here in Montreal.

This book comes from his heart, his solid faith in God, his own family's experience, and his vast experience as a physician.

I pray that *Made to Live* will be a source of inspiration, information, and encouragement to the reader.

—Rev. Knut Kollmar
Lasalle, Quebec

In *Made to Live*, Dr. Paul Saba has provided a timely reminder of the underlying principles of medicine, which are to heal, promote health, and alleviate suffering, and to resist the temptation of killing the patient. Outlining his personal, family, and professional struggles to resist pressure coming from within the medical profession to take human life rather than preserve and cherish it, he provides valuable insight into the dangers posed to true medicine by the corrupting influence of the spread of euthanasia and assisted suicide. With reference to the history of the euthanasia movement, he shows that it is fundamentally opposed to the principles of medicine.

—Dr. Gordon Macdonald
CEO, Care Not Killing, London, UK

In my country, the suicide rates are the highest in Europe, and active euthanasia has been legalized since 2002. I have experienced how the law works personally, and I have tried to warn other countries not to choose the path we have chosen in my country.

Dr. Paul Saba experienced the technological revolution personally, leading him to rethink his role as a physician, but also as a husband, as a father, and as a family member connected to the society around him.

In *Made to Live*, Dr. Saba describes the personal journey that has led him to oppose strongly the euthanasia laws giving physicians the legal power to choose between life and death. However, for him it is utterly clear that physicians shouldn't be in the business of killing, since the role of the physician is to give hope and to protect life. I endorse this book, and I do hope that many people will read it. Choosing death is definitely not the right solution to face the urgent problems in this century. We are indeed all *Made to Live*.

—Tom Mortier, Ph.D.
Lecturer, Author, & Anti-Euthanasia Activist, Belgium

Dr. Saba brings to this crucial debate a physician's mind, a researcher's eye, a passion for justice, a father's heart, and a life of experience in caring for vulnerable people—not just in Canada, but in resource-poor settings in Central America, Asia, Africa, and the Middle East. He has produced a book which is a masterly blend of hard evidence, sound argument, human compassion, ethical reflection, and good medicine. Laws allowing assisted suicide or euthanasia are unnecessary (because better alternatives exist), dangerous (because of their risk to the vulnerable), and morally wrong (contrary to all historic codes of medical ethics). Human beings are "made to live" and real "death with dignity" is achieved through care that addresses people's physical, psychological, and spiritual needs. Such a path is more costly, both financially and emotionally, than dispensing lethal drugs, but the mark of a truly just and compassionate society is one in which the strong make sacrifices for those who are sick, weak and vulnerable rather than sacrificing them.

—Dr. Peter Saunders
CEO, International Christian Medical and Dental Association
(ICMDA)
Chair, End of Life Care Europe (ELCE)

Dr. Paul Saba shares his personal experiences and family story, opening our hearts to his personal human experience to understand how killing is not a solution to human problems.

I consider Dr. Paul Saba to truly be a canary in the coal mine, alerting the world about the fatal flaws associated with euthanasia and assisted suicide.

This book is an incredible addition to the arsenal of data and stories upholding the value of human life and enunciating why killing people is not only bad public policy but simply wrong.

—Alex Schadenberg
Executive Director & International Chair, Euthanasia Prevention Coalition

Made to Live penetrates through the haze of the hype and lays out the facts you need to know. Read this book in order to educate yourself about "Medical Aid in Dying" before it is presented as an option to you, your loved ones, or your friends. This is a riveting must-read that you won't be able to put down.

—David Stevens, M.D., M.A. (Ethics)
CEO Emeritus, Christian Medical & Dental Associations

Having lived in a wheelchair for more than fifty years, I personally understand the difficult challenges of living with a disability. I have spent the majority of my life educating policy makers and well-meaning physicians about the dangers of physician-assisted suicide and euthanasia. People with disabilities need advocates like Dr. Paul Saba, who personally knows that the hard choice to help someone live with disability is the right choice, no matter the cost to society or caregivers. *Made to Live: A Physician's Journey to Save Life* is an honest, heart-wrenching personal journey of a father and a physician proving that life is worth saving, and no one is "better off dead."

—Joni Eareckson Tada
Founder & CEO, Joni and Friends International Disability Center

MADE TO LIVE

A Physician's Journey
to Save Life

PAUL SABA M.D.

MADE TO LIVE
Copyright © 2020 by Paul Saba M.D.

Scripture marked NIV taken from The Holy Bible, New International Version®, NIV® Copyright ©1973, 1978, 1984, 2011 by Biblica, Inc.® Used by permission. All rights reserved worldwide. • Scripture marked NKJV taken from the New King James Version®, Copyright © 1982 by Thomas Nelson, Inc. Used by permission. All rights reserved.

The views and opinions expressed in this publication belong solely to the author and do not reflect those of Word Alive Press or any of its employees.

Printed in Canada

ISBN: 978-1-4866-1922-1
eBook ISBN: 978-1-4866-1923-8

Word Alive Press
119 De Baets Street Winnipeg, MB R2J 3R9
www.wordalivepress.ca

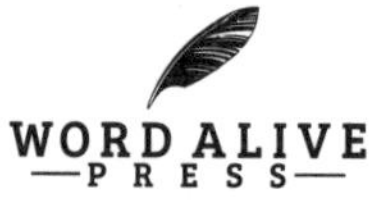

Cataloguing in Publication information can be obtained from Library and Archives Canada.

---

[1] Available at https://www.sefaria.org/Mishnah_Sanhedrin.4.5?lang=bi.

Contents

ACKNOWLEDGEMENTS

I would like to thank first and foremost my wife Marisa, who has been a great support during my long absences as a physician caring for my patients. She has had to endure my endless conferences, media interviews, and battles: to save St. Joseph's Hospital (now called Lachine Hospital), and the costly fight against euthanasia and assisted suicide. My children have been amazing in their insights and patience. They have given me far more than I can ever give them. I thank my wife and children for their love.

I want to acknowledge the love, support, and inspiration of my parents, John and Rhoda, who both showed me in tangible ways what real love and sacrifice mean.

I want to thank my patients, who have been courageous in battling against the adversity of illness and disabilities, and who have inspired me to fight on their behalf.

I want to thank Dr. Francis Humphrey, who lived with ALS for fifteen years with his wife Daria faithfully by his side. He wrote *Origins and Redemption*, about the science of God's creation of the world, typing one letter at a time—with a pencil-end secured to his hand—until he needed to be connected to a respirator. He continued to "write" inspiring sermons employing his eyes and a computer while on his breathing machine for the rest of his life, which ended peacefully at home from natural causes.[2]

I want to thank Lisa D'Amico, who, despite her disability and her challenges, has had the courage and perseverance to carry on. I also want to thank her lawyer, Gerard Samet, for staying by her side.

I want to thank my lawyer, Natalia Manole, who has stayed by me through thick and thin during the gargantuan court battles against both the Quebec and Canadian governments, who have been steamrollers in their attempts to silence any opposition to assisted suicide and euthanasia.

I want to thank my sister Georgina, who has been an invaluable help when I needed support "at the last minute" at press conferences or media events.

I want to thank the media, who have allowed me to be heard, although in limited ways because of the perceived popularity of euthanasia and assisted suicide.

I want to thank all my family and friends for helping me with my many causes.

I want to thank my daughter Jessica, whose painting of our family entitled "Made to Live" inspired the title and theme of this book.

I want to thank my son John-Anthony, whose original cover design was inspired by a woven heart of yarn that reminds me of King David's verse from Psalm 139:13 (NIV), *"For you created my inmost being; you knit me together in my mother's womb."* It reminds

---

[2] "Choosing to Live with Good Care and Dignity: A Case of Severe Amyotrophic Lateral Sclerosis (ALS)," *CoalitionMD.org*, June 5, 2013 (http://coalitionmd.org/en/choosing-to-live-with-good-care-and-dignity-a-case-of-severe-amyotrophic-lateral-sclerosis-als/); "Doctor Opposes Assisted Suicide Bill," *CBC.ca*, June 5, 2013 (https://www.cbc.ca/news/canada/doctor-opposes-assisted-suicide-bill-1.430169); Anne LeClair, "Dying ALS Patient and His Doctors Speak Out against Assisted Suicide," *Global News*, June 5, 2013 (https://globalnews.ca/news/618291/dying-als-patient-and-his-doctors-speak-out-against-assisted-suicide/).

us of our humanness and value, starting from the moment of conception. The heart symbolizes life.

I want to thank my daughter Eliana, who contributed greatly to the last chapter and challenges us to invest in the lives of future generations.

I want to thank my content editor Peter Stockland for his insights, encouragement, and comments in helping me bring this book to publication.

I want to thank the Word Alive Press team for their professionalism.

Finally, I want to thank Jesus for His example of selfless love, hope and caring.

Introduction

The purpose of this book is to remind everyone how precious life is. I do mean everyone: politicians who might be moved to act on its message, journalists who might communicate at least some of its ideas and arguments, and perhaps most of all, ordinary readers who might feel doubtful, confused—even misled—by the diminishing value placed on life that has come into our culture in recent years.

Through my training as a doctor, my experience as a husband and father, and my reflections on my deepest ideals, I want to join my voice with those who reject the new mythology that life is only a disposable commodity to be used up and tossed into the recycling bin. No! We are made to live. Now, more than ever, we need to re-learn that truth.

The book that follows flows most directly from my research and engagement during ten years of standing against so-called Medical Aid in Dying (MAiD), which is now law in my home province of Quebec and across Canada. In reality, though, it goes back much further to a gut feeling that prematurely ending human life under the pretext of giving medical "assistance" is a terrible thing. I instinctively knew it was wrong to kill our fellow human beings, even with state sanctioning, in a hospital, clinic, or doctor's office.

Support for that instinctive sense comes from studying the history of euthanasia itself. We can go back to the middle of the last century when it was practiced in Germany in a terrible systematic form. Or we can go back a few millennia to the development of the Hippocratic Oath, which was expressly crafted to forbid medical killing. In either case, and all those in between, we see the wrongness of government (in whatever form) sanctioning the killing of citizens. Reflecting on that brings me to reflect on what has happened to me personally to make me value life so very much. It makes me further reflect that while we cannot let go of political engagement, and (when possible) still need to take on legal battles such as those I have tried to wage, our primary mission must be as witnesses to the truth of life as a precious gift. We mirror for those around us the conviction that we are made to live.

Of course, we all know each of us will die. We might wish to deny it. We might seek to delay it as long as we can. But in our hearts, we know its inevitability. As a son, I watched my own father's health deteriorate, and that was a deep personal shock to me. As a physician, from my time as a medical student through to my many years of practice, I've regularly seen people dying. Some I would come to know well; others I met only through the emergency room when trying to resuscitate them. Our mortality is inseparable from our humanity.

Yet the whole purpose of any physician is to try to save life. It is to try to turn the inevitable around and see people going on to live. Often, we succeed. Other times, we fail. But state-sanctioned killing is very different from doctors falling short of continuing the precious gift of life. Government using healthcare professionals to carry out medically administered death goes against my very sense of why I became a doctor.

Here in Quebec, when the provincial government first opened up a consultation about what would come to be euphemistically called MAiD, I was shocked. I could not believe we were opening up that debate. At the time, they were considering only euthanasia. There wasn't even a discussion of assisted suicide—that came later.

I knew I had to get involved in the consultation. During my research for the first brief that I submitted, I discovered only a few other countries had opened the door that way: Belgium and the Netherlands, Luxembourg in a slightly different fashion, and Switzerland, which had assisted suicide. Given the small number of countries involved, and their all being small countries as well, I was convinced that as the debate and consultation process took place, a large number of Canadian physicians would stand up against it. I was surprised, and greatly dismayed, when that didn't happen.

Then the Quebec government made clear it was moving ahead with MAiD regardless of what the consultation process determined people wanted. The media got involved, inundating people with stories of those who wanted to die rather than endure agonizing suffering. That's when I started looking at it. I asked of myself and others: "Well, is this true? Can we, in fact, not take care of human suffering? Can we not provide support and care whether it's psychological, medical, or medication?" As I did my research, I realized that yes, we could. So why were we going down the road to MAiD?

I became more and more convinced that there was an interest within the government to promote it. There were groups of activists committed to the whole idea of euthanasia and assisted suicide—what's now called MAiD. I learned that there was historical precedent for this—it wasn't something that just came out of nowhere. The desire to take life when we believe we can no longer control it has been going on for thousands of years. The difference is that historically we have differentiated between those who are killers and those who are healers.

Even knowing where Quebec's consultation process was going, I submitted a number of briefs to both the Quebec and Canadian governments. I submitted to the Quebec government in 2010 and again in 2012. Then in 2016, I submitted two briefs to the Canadian government. When that seemed—pardon the pun—a dead end, I met with some lawyers who agreed to take on a legal challenge case because we saw the government was clearly going to legislate MAiD.

In May 2014, approximately a week before the Quebec government's legislation, we launched a temporary injunction to try to stop it. It was ignored. We weren't able to get the judges to agree to it. But we continued in the courts and were temporarily able to stop the law. We even had the federal government on our side for a while because we were able to make the case that there was a federal prohibition on killing, and that the Quebec government could not constitutionally pass a law that infringed on federal laws.

Then the federal government did an about-face. The Prime Minister went public before we went to court. The federal Attorney General also did an about-face. Quebec challenged our standing to stop the legislation. We thought about taking a case about public interference to the Supreme Court, but our lawyers told us that since the Supreme Court had already ruled unanimously in favor of MAiD, our chances were very slim regardless of whether there was political interference. We decided to go back to Superior Court and continue our challenge there on different matters.

The Attorney General of Quebec wrote in their court proceedings that I was not allowed to present my arguments against assisted suicide and euthanasia because I was against it.

The Attorney General of Canada agreed. Their argument was that since I was "not a supporter or defender of medical aid in dying"[3] I could not object to it. Their argument made no sense, because if I had no opinions about assisted suicide and euthanasia, I would not have been challenging the law. On the other hand, if I was for euthanasia and assisted suicide (as were both governments), it appears that I would have been permitted to present any arguments in favour of MAiD. This goes against my fundamental Canadian Charter Rights and Freedoms, which include freedom of thought, opinion, and expression. This reminds me of George Orwell's classic novel *Nineteen Eighty-Four* where members of the ruling class use brazenly misleading terminology including double speak (MAiD), double think (killing is medical), and mind control (you can only think what the state wants you to think). Even in Canada, you're only allowed to think and express what the state wants you to. To drive the point home, the judge even forced me to pay court costs. This means I had to pay the court costs incurred by the governments, both provincial and federal, despite this being a public interest case, despite my having no financial interest whatsoever in the case, and despite my purpose being to save lives from needlessly being thrown away.

I'm not even allowed to speak against MAiD in court because… I'm against it. I've always thought that's what courts are for: opposing sides present their best arguments, and the rule of law prevails. Sometimes I wonder if that's still true in Canada. Have we really come to a place where we're not even allowed to think differently than what the state mandates? Are we not allowed to express our opinions if they go against what the state expresses? That's not the Canada I remember growing up in.

---

[3] Attorney General of Quebec, "Motion to Dismiss," April 20, 2017: Dr Saba c. PGQ-PGC/Dossier C.S. 500-17-082567-143, paragraphs 29–31.

It has been a long fight. It has often been a tiring fight. Still, I believe that in retrospect, history will look on us favourably and say we were fighting for life—fighting for humankind. Regardless of the outcome, I want to continue to help people become aware of the myths, manipulations, and marketing of MAiD. I want to continue making the case for why it doesn't belong in our culture at all, and certainly doesn't belong in our healthcare system.

As a doctor, I know just how dangerous it is to make the killing of patients part of the healthcare system, part of what we call medicine or medical aid. Physicians are not God. When doctors give a patient a diagnosis, we can be wrong. In fact, errors in diagnosis for severe, life-threatening conditions can be as high as twenty percent.[4]

Recently, a man came to me with a cough, a cold. He had a chest x-ray. According to the radiologist's reading of the chest film, my patient most probably had lung cancer. I sat down with him and said: "We need to do a scan right away. We need to get you to see a specialist. We need to do a bronchoscopy…."

Here was his answer: "Dr. Saba, I know you're against euthanasia and assisted suicide, but you know what? I don't necessarily agree with you. If I'm going to die, if my time is up…."

I replied, "No, no. You have to go through the process because this is only a preliminary diagnosis. Even if it is lung cancer, that is treatable today. There are new treatments. It may not even be lung cancer."

I spoke to the radiologist, who said, "We're not sure what it is. We don't know if it's lymphoma, which would be highly treatable. It may be something else."

Here was an intelligent, well-informed man, an engineer, who thought he had a cold, then thought he had cancer, and could have

---

[4] M.L. Graber, R.M. Wachter, & C.K. Cassel (2012), "Bringing Diagnosis into the Quality and Safety Equations," *Journal of the American Medical Association* 308, no. 12 (2012): 1211–1212.

resigned himself to MAiD before he even knew what we were dealing with, or what the treatment might be. He could have given up hope while the situation was still filled with hope. That power to move people to give up is one of the dangerous and misleading aspects of medically assisted death. However, I was able to get his attention and persuade him that the situation was hopeful and that he should get investigated and treated. In the end, the patient called me in the summer of 2019 to thank me for this medical cure. He had finally been diagnosed with Hodgkin's lymphoma, which is a condition that is highly curable with proper medical treatment.

By contrast, hope is a one of the most powerful forces for good medical care. I am a Christian. I believe God can, and does, work miracles in our lives and in the world around us. But I am a Christian doctor, and so I also believe medicine must be grounded in solid science, in what research and experience teach us about how the body works and heals. When I say hope is a powerful force for health, I mean the way it counsels us to patience, to seeing processes through, and to regarding every step as part of the great gift of being made for life.

I've seen confirmation of my Christian beliefs, and evidence for medical science, throughout my career as a doctor, whether in Quebec, Canada, the United States, or in Bangladesh, Somalia, and the Ivory Coast. I've seen it most profoundly in my life as a husband and father.

Before my daughter Jessica was born, we were told at twenty and again at twenty-four weeks of pregnancy that there was a serious problem. On the ultrasound, they saw she had a thick neck and a defective heart. They said it was Down syndrome, and that we should "look at all of our options," which really meant having an abortion. In Canada, we have the "option" to abort Down syndrome babies—along with every other baby until the moment of delivery.

We immediately said: "No. We're not going there." We prayed to God, "Please fix the heart. Please, God, make sure it's not Down syndrome." We prayed, "Please don't take our daughter." Well, it wasn't Down syndrome, and we're thankful, despite the fact that children who have Down's have wonderful lives. We know parents of Down syndrome kids, and they are as happy as any parents can be.

There was a new procedure to repair Jessica's heart, and it was successful. So she, who might have been an abortion "option," is now a loving, active, happy member of our family. She reminds us every day what a precious gift life is.

In fact, I asked her one day to draw me a picture of our family the way she sees us. Partly, I wanted to keep her busy, and at the same time keep her off the computer and the Internet. Of course, she went to the computer and drew the picture using a computer program. She drew us as a family, with her picture and her name larger than the other names. And then she put a title on it: Made to Live. I didn't even suggest those words to her. She just wrote them above us as a family. I looked at the title, and I looked at that little person in that little picture, and then I looked at her. I said, "Jessica, you were made to live. We're all made to live."

That, really, is my purpose in writing this book: to keep people on the path of life that even little children know in their hearts we're made to walk down.

Chapter 1

The Worth of a Human Life

All of us live lives filled with multiple roles. Some of the roles that comprise my own life are husband, father, physician, citizen. Of course, I'm also a son, a brother, an uncle… the list could stretch on for a page, or even pages.

A key lesson I've learned in the effort to fight for life—not merely to fight *against* euthanasia—is the way in which these many roles overlap and connect to support each other like the parts of a bridge. They make us identifiable as individuals. Each role contributes something to us being a whole human person. They explain both the how and the why of us being made to live. In my Christian understanding, they are the evidence of God creating us and, following that, living on Earth in human form for our salvation.

Though obviously I would argue it can help, you don't need Judeo-Christian faith to see how our many-sided and interwoven lives reveal euthanasia as a terrible social and spiritual misdiagnosis of the human condition. It is based, after all, on the assumption that radical autonomy is our natural state.

For euthanasia to prevail in a society, whether a democratic one such as Canada or a totalitarian fascist state such as Nazi Germany, a substantial percentage of the population must become convinced that our existence and our value is based on mental or physical perfection. This was the Nazi thinking expressed by the words "Lebensunwertes Leben" (lives unworthy of life). Conversely, only certain lives are deemed worthy of life.

A son described to me the emotional distress he felt watching his mother decline physically, yet not receiving adequate pain control for her osteoarthritis. Many times the family was called to her bedside because her "time was at the end," but she would then rebound back. She had become a burden and an inconvenience that wore on the emotions of the family, some of whom had to travel a distance to visit her. She finally died after several years. He would have preferred a "planned death" with the family around at a specific time.

Fabian Stahle, in a 2017 *Journal of Ethics in Mental Health* article, describes the process of moral disengagement that allows people to kill fellow human beings through euthanasia and assisted suicide:

> This way of emphasizing the sick person's limitations and reduced possibilities for an independent life is tantamount to dehumanization. It is the degradation of a human being into a sub-human object with a lower protection value, in order to make it easier to participate in the person's death. … One can also blame the patient by emphasizing the emotional and/or financial burden he or she is causing the relatives and society at large. In this way, the patient is declared guilty and sentenced to death due to all the inconvenience, discomfort, and dismay the person is causing.[5]

---

[5] Fabian Stahle, "Moral Disengagement—Mechanisms Propelling the Euthanasia/PAS Movement," *Journal of Ethics in Mental Health* 10 (2017): 1–15.

We are simply like random containers on a grocery store shelf, stamped with best-before and dispose-of-after dates. When we're gone, we're gone, and fresh product will replace us.

The multiplicities we experience in our own lives discredit the logic and expose the mythical basis of such a claim. When we're gone, those with whom our lives were interwoven remain behind. If our lives are ended prematurely by an overt act of medicalized killing, all those we've been connected to know in their hearts (even if ideology prevents them speaking it on their lips) that we have lived less than the full life available to us. It implies that we are a replaceable product that has been removed, not human beings made to live and made to be connected to each other to the natural end of life.

There are multiple tragic effects from the discredited, discreditable, and mythical aspects of euthanasia seeping into and saturating a society. One that affects me most profoundly is the way it distorts the meaning of medicine. I'm not alone in being affected that way.

Even doctors who profess neutrality about the legal changes that permitted euthanasia in Canada and Quebec will frequently acknowledge—and have acknowledged to me—that it has no place in the medical system. It is not medicine. It is the opposite of medicine. Doctors are not trained, and very few enter the profession, to intentionally kill.

But there's another, deeper reason. Every doctor who practices knows that virtually every procedure we do has built into it the risk of misdiagnosis. If euthanasia itself is a social misdiagnosis, what are its tragic implications for doctors who are always working under the weight of the risk of a medical misdiagnosis in a culture of intentional killing?

It's not that doctors are bad at their jobs. Not at all. It's the reality that no one has perfect judgement, and medicine is much more about judgement than it is about machine-like perfect knowledge.

I have a patient who, in 2004, was told he had lung cancer. He says he would have asked for euthanasia then if it had been available—he would have ended his life years ago if he could have. He had only a lung infection. It was discovered after they took him to the operating room, removed the lung, and did a biopsy right there. He's alive today. The only reason he still shares his life with the interwoven lives around him is because euthanasia wasn't available at that time.

Yet today euthanasia *is* available. And we can see from that one example what a dangerous option it has given people. Killing isn't a risk or an option. It's an intention. Its entire purpose is as a lethal weapon that people can use at any time to kill themselves, or can require doctors to make use of to carry out state-sanctioned killing using lethal injections.

What is the effect going to be on our collective future as Canadians, and on our lives with their multiplicity of roles? For one, it will sink us deeper and deeper into the mythology of radical autonomy. We often think of errors—or misdiagnoses—as things that happen once and then belong to the past. But we know from our own experience there are certain wrongs that must be repeated over and over because stopping them requires admitting and accepting the full guilt for them as offences.

Slavery was one of them. Abortion is another. To admit now that abortion is wrong would be to confess at least social culpability in the killing of millions upon millions of unborn children since the procedure was "medicalized" and legalized in the 1960s and 1970s. It would be to suffer something of what the post-war German people experienced at the end of the Holocaust. Our current myth of radical autonomy, and its use to justify euthanasia, is leading us down an analogous historical path. It is leading us to deny that what makes us human is that we are made to live.

To live our lives in a multiplicity of roles means, of course, that we live them out through a wide variety of experiences. As a physician, I have lived and worked in many different cultural contexts. I've experienced many different ways of living. I try to make sense of those experiences for their own richness, but also for the way they affect who I am today.

Though I've spent the majority of my medical practice here in Canada, I spent close to a dozen years working in the United States, both in my residency and internal medicine practice (for which I am Board Certified in the U.S.). I worked in the emergency room in North Carolina at Duke Medical Center for three years and in Massachusetts. I've worked in Africa. I've worked in Bangladesh. I worked in Lebanon during my last year of residency in internal medicine.

The universal theme is that human life is valuable wherever you are. Whether you're in Africa, whether you're in Bangladesh, whether you're in North America, human life is valuable. In my experiences meeting other doctors, the vast majority of physicians I've met, the vast majority of all the people I've met, express strong commitment to the value of human life.

Yet Canada—where I live, and where I was born—has chosen to completely disregard that commitment to human life, which I've heard everywhere else I've been in the world. We have a universal healthcare system, which is a way to provide accessibility to everyone. As a country we profess—and I believe sincerely—that society must take care of the weak, the sick, the vulnerable, those who need help and support when they cannot help and support themselves.

At the same time, we become champions for using that medical system to end people's lives. To me, it's what we mean when we call something schizophrenic. Now, when you deal with people who have schizophrenia, you don't condemn them. They see a different world. You try to help them. We have to help people see that euthanasia itself, and the ideology underlying it, goes against medical care. We have to find a way to get people back to reality.

Right now, we've lost our grip on reality. We as Canadians, from ordinary people to people with real political power, are saying it makes sense if a person wants to end their life because they can't take life anymore. No. No. It doesn't! Life is valuable. There is a purpose in your life—in every life.

Acknowledging life's value, acknowledging life's purpose, does not deny the reality of suffering. My job involves treating people who are suffering. I know they are suffering. And, as a physician, sometimes I have to communicate bad news to them. I have to explain to my patients their options for treatment. I always try to portray a hopeful attitude. I try to help them see there is much they can still do with their lives, that ending life isn't the best— much less only—option. I say, "Write. Paint. Draw. Tell stories. Be with those whom you are connected with, and who are connected to you, until the natural end of your life."

In many ways, the worst aspect of euthanasia's social and spiritual misdiagnosis of our human condition is that it denies our calling to help and support those around us right to the very end. We need to help. We need to support. Whether the suffering is physical or psychological, whether it's cancer or schizophrenia, we do wrong to bring life to an end prematurely. Why? Because, just as doctors can misdiagnose and deliver a wrong prognosis, we cannot humanly know what or when the end of a life will be.

Those words are not abstractions. I experience them regularly as a doctor. But my most powerful experience of them was as a father.

When I got the news about my unborn daughter Jessica's medical conditions, I felt devastated. It was as if the floor had fallen from under my feet. I reached out to other doctors to better understand the medical options. My wife and I contacted our pastor and asked friends to pray for us.

We prayed that the situation would change. We prayed that Jessica would not have the heart condition. When we realized that the heart condition was real, severe, and wasn't going away, we prayed that the physicians caring for her would successfully treat her condition so that she would survive.

When my wife approached the delivery date, she was asked how aggressively to save Jessica if she was born severely deformed with little chance of survival. Marisa courageously responded, "I have done everything to come this far, and you do everything you need to do to keep her alive."

In order to ensure the best chances of survival for Jessica, a caesarean birth was planned with a full team of specialists standing by. However, Jessica had her own time schedule. Six days prior to the planned birth, Marisa started to experience birthing contractions. Jessica was not going to wait for the planned arrival date.

Marisa was having so much pain, the obstetrician decided to perform the caesarean section late at night. It was done just in the nick of time. The uterine wall was paper thin and coming apart at the incision line. Both Marisa and Jessica's lives would have been endangered if the procedure had been delayed for even a few more minutes.

Jessica was born and immediately taken under the care of the paediatric intensive care team. Just before she was transferred to the Montreal Children's Hospital, Marisa held Jessica briefly in her arms and encouraged her: "You fight, little girl—you fight."

While at the Children's Hospital I stayed at Jessica's bedside. I sang songs and held her hand. I prayed constantly for her survival. I begged God not to take my precious daughter away from me. I prayed that God would make a way for her to survive. I would have given the world to keep her in my life. Marisa joined me a few days later, as she was slowly recovering from her caesarean section. Jessica was continually on oxygen and connected to an intravenous tube so that she could receive lifesaving medication to keep her fetal heart circulation intact.

At six days old, Jessica underwent a cardiac intervention. The cardiologist was surprised that the valve needing to be opened actually had a pinhole of 0.2 mm, which allowed him to thread the catheter and open her heart valve. The procedure is called a balloon valvuloplasty. If there was no opening in the valve, there was a risk of perforating her heart, which would have meant almost an immediate death.

The unexpected pinhole opening reminded my wife Marisa of one of her favorite songs: "God Will Make a Way." Gradually Jessica improved. At eleven months old, she underwent a second procedure. Today, her paediatric cardiologist says that if he didn't know Jessica's cardiac history, he would never guess that she had a severe cardiac anomaly. Developmentally she has excelled in all areas of her life.

My daughter's precarious birth taught me, in a way even my years of medical training and experience could not, that every life is valuable. No one can guarantee outcomes. We may have some ideas of the future, but they are most often illusory. What is real is the loving support of friends and family that surrounded us during our ordeal. It was our greatest need during a time of such uncertainty. It is the greatest need all of us have in the multiple roles we play in our own lives, and in the lives of those around us.

That's why I'm able to say to those struggling through serious health challenges, and for whom the outlook appears dim: "Never give up on life, even as your life draws to an end. You are worthy of life. You are made to live."

CHAPTER 2

HOW I LEARNED TO VALUE LIFE

I did not grow up as a little boy dreaming of becoming a doctor who would spend a great deal of money waging a court battle against his own government to stop the state from allowing people to be killed by the publicly funded healthcare system. In fact, as a young man (and for quite a few years after I was no longer such a young man), I was too busy enjoying my life to think about becoming personally involved in such a fight. Thinking about it, though, I see in hindsight that getting involved as deeply as I did must have been influenced by the ethic of the family into which I was born, and which led me into medicine in the first place.

When my wife Marisa told Jessica at our darkest hour, "You fight, little girl," she was passing along the spirit that infuses and inspires our family, too. We are made to live, and sometimes living requires standing up and fighting as best you can for what you most deeply believe.

My life in recent years has been lived out in the battle over Medical Aid in Dying, in newspaper stories and TV interviews, and in court cases where we tasted victory and then had it taken from us. But it's also been lived less than three kilometres from where I was born to a family of Lebanese-Syrian descent, almost in the shadow of the old Dominion Bridge works in Lachine.

My father owned his own clothing business in Lachine. His parents immigrated from Lebanon in 1898, while my mother's parents were also immigrants from Lebanon and Syria. I remind people that the Lebanese are descendants of the Phoenician trading empire and invented the Western alphabet. I tell my children their ancestry is one-eighth Syrian, three-eighths Lebanese, and half Italian because my wife's family is Italian.

When I was growing up, neither my dad nor my grandparents could get jobs at Dominion Bridge. Dominion Bridge did not hire immigrants or their immediate descendents. In fact, my family couldn't even get a loan from the bank, so they had to borrow from their French Canadian neighbours. After I became a doctor, I met someone who remembered a story being passed down from her great-grandfather—her family was angry because the Saba family paid back the money they borrowed too quickly, depriving her family of interest payments they had hoped to earn.

In classic immigrant fashion, the Sabas began to build housing for their French Canadian neighbours. They lost a lot of it during the Depression because they still had to pay taxes on buildings where the renters had no money. My grandparents didn't have the heart to throw people out of their apartments and replace them with people who could pay the rent, so they took the losses and lost many of the buildings.

When I was a child growing up in one of those buildings, my siblings and I would play with families that were Italian or French or English-speaking because the houses shared a common backyard, and my mom built a large sandbox that everybody could share and play in. She was an American citizen, born in the United States, who married my dad, came to Canada, and raised our family. She served on the Home and School Association while raising four kids, trying to learn French, and writing letters to whomever she could protesting violence on television. She has always had a very strong Christian faith, but she had trouble finding a church she felt really taught true Biblical principles. For a while, she was a Sunday school teacher at a United Church, but then they changed the curriculum in a way that questioned the Bible.

My mom told the pastor, "I can't teach this."

He said, "Teach what you want, plus teach that."

She said, "I can't do both. I can't pretend." My mom resigned from the United Church, pulled us out of the Sunday school program, and "home churched" us for a while after that.

Those Christian principles, and the principles of that immigrant life, formed who I am. In my late teens, I went off to university and started questioning everything, became an agnostic, and lived in uncertainty for a while. In medical school, they called me Disco Duck. I never missed an opportunity to have a good time. I got my heart broken, and I broke other hearts. Being a medical student carries a certain prestige, a certain attractiveness. But I always felt alone. I suffered from terrible feelings of loneliness.

As I've gone through life, that period has helped me understand how desperately people will seek to fight the loneliness they feel in so many different ways. In the previous chapter, I described Medical Aid in Dying as a misdiagnosis of our human condition. One of the symptoms I believe it misreads so dangerously is physical suffering where the pain is really spiritual, psychological, and emotional—a consuming fear born of awful loneliness. It ends up confusing death with relief.

I was certainly suffering from a degree of that loneliness when I went to Hawaii as a young doctor seeking another experience, another opportunity to meet someone who might break my heart, whose heart I might break, or who might—just might—make me whole. Instead, I met God. And I met God because I saw a sign.

Literally. I kept seeing a sign that said there was going to be a beach service on Sunday at a particular location.

I kept running into that sign, almost tripping over it. I later discovered there was actually only one sign, but I was… busy… going here and there, so I thought the sign was everywhere.

I decided to go to a service at the hotel instead. The pastor there was a reformed drug addict who said, "There's someone you're looking for. That person is Jesus."

I said to myself, "This guy knows." He knew what he was talking about. He was really down to earth. Other people had told me I was going to Hell, but I wasn't sure there was a Heaven so I wasn't too worried about Hell. My philosophy was that I might as well enjoy the party while I was on Earth.

I debated going to talk to the pastor afterward, but, in the end, pride got in the way. I told myself I was spending a lot of money to be there; I might as well enjoy myself. I headed to the beach and happened to see the most beautiful woman I'd ever seen in my whole life. It was like a sunbeam was shining down on her.

I said to myself, "That is what I'm missing." I said to God: "We'll finish our conversation later. I've got to take care of this immediate situation here. This is an emergency."

So, I went into the water and swam toward her. I was careful not to look like I was accosting her—I was just a guy out swimming—but as I got close, I said, "Isn't it a beautiful day?"

She replied, "It's a wonderful day." I knew I had made contact, and we started a conversation. I made small talk, asked how her day was going, what she'd been doing. She said, "Well, I started off today praying and asking God to bring me somebody I could witness to."

It was like checkmate. I said, "Well, I guess I'm that person." I found out she was married, which was disappointing, and her husband was right there on the beach, which was about as disappointing as it could get.

But we talked, and she really answered the questions I wanted to ask that pastor.

I didn't buy into Christianity being happy, happy, happy. People always told me, "You'll be so happy," but I wasn't happy and couldn't imagine Christianity would change that. She told me very honestly, "Some of my worst days have been as a Christian. But I can call on Jesus to help me and to get me through the day." It was such a real experience to talk to somebody who expressed Christianity as a struggle, as a journey, but not something that had to be faced alone. It became real to me. And I knew what I needed in my life was Jesus—He was what I was missing.

Later, there was a brief beach service in front of the Hilton Hotel. A pastor prayed with me and I accepted Christ. My life changed, and my way of looking at life started to change. I didn't know which church to go to, but I started meeting people and going to various Christian denominations and my faith grew.

I was in my thirties then. Did I become this perfect specimen of virtue overnight? No. There were lots of things I had to deal with and change in my life. I thought God would bring me a wife right away. It wasn't to be—I didn't get married until I was fifty. I often joke that the good-looking guys got married first and I had to wait my turn. There was a long, dry season in terms of waiting to find the right spouse. It was often a difficult journey.

Did I always act as a Christian? No. But I got better at it. Not better in terms of this perfect human person, but a person whose faith grew. And I think I became a kinder person. I also became more engaged socially.

What really enticed me was the social gospel, Christ's call to help our fellow human beings. That's the thing that always amazed me about Christ. He healed people. He fed people. He was constantly talking about our need to do better, to do more for our fellow human beings. And it didn't become just an obligation—it was something that I enjoyed. When I got involved in working in the developing world, I felt fulfilled. When I spent more time with my patients and really found the problem, I felt fulfilled. Getting socially involved in fighting for free medications for those who couldn't afford to pay for them, fighting for the community hospital: they were tough battles. But I felt like I was doing something. And I consider that a whole part of the way God has changed my heart. I was no longer the Disco Duck.

My mom visits people endlessly in hospitals, in nursing homes. She has all these relationships with the people she cares for. She brings casseroles to people twenty years younger than she is. And I think this kind of service is what we miss because we've gotten into such a mindset of me, me, me; busy, busy, busy. By the way, my mom is ninety-three years old.

We don't see the value of stopping and taking care of each other. It's not profitable. Can't make money doing that. Time is money. Well, time is for people. People sometimes say to me, "Well, it's easy for you, Dr. Saba. You're a doctor and you have a good income." I know that. But I don't have to spend my money in court battles against my own government to stop the state from allowing people to be killed by the publicly funded healthcare system. I do it, though. Not because I'm this perfect human being. But because I believe in it—because I believe it is what God gave me life to do.

When we become engaged in life, when we help people, it breathes life into us. God made us for that. He gave us a purpose. Jesus gave us instructions to feed the hungry, to clothe the naked to give, to heal… He instructed his disciples to do that, and we are his disciples.

There's a Bible verse that says, *"He has put eternity in their hearts"* (Ecclesiastes 3:11, NKJV). So even for those who don't have a confessing faith in Christ, God has put a sense of purpose in their heart. He made us to live so we're not fulfilled by eating more, having faster cars, bigger houses. We need the basics, and we have a responsibility to ensure that everybody has the basics. But at the same time, those things don't satisfy the heart. God satisfies the heart. Thank God I saw that sign.

CHAPTER 3
PATIENTS ARE PERSONS

Practicing medicine can become very mechanical. You're in the hospital. You're working with patients. You're part of a resuscitation team, especially as an intern. There are regular steps you follow to bring people back. Circulation, airway, and breathing are part of the American Heart Association's algorithm to try to get the heart restarted during cardiac arrest. You see life and death in the minutes you have to work on someone until, at a certain point, you have to call it quits. Some people come back. Some don't. The process hasn't changed dramatically in the years I've practiced other than in the medications we use.

But what can feel like a routine doesn't change the dramatic effect it has on people, on the families you have to meet and talk to, which is always the hardest part. Then you get to know at least a little bit—sometimes a lot—about who this person was. It's not just a body with a heart that stopped, a body that stopped breathing. There's a whole story with a human person behind it.

The reality of the humanity in every person's story is why I still remember the sense of personal defeat and, yes, loss I felt at Framingham Union Hospital long ago, when, as an intern, I was called at around 3 a.m. to try to resuscitate someone who could not be revived. We did everything properly. During the debrief afterward, my colleagues on the code team with me said "It's not your fault. You did everything." But it still stays in my mind as a failure.

Why? Because, before medical practice becomes mechanical and routine, you start off with the sense you can accomplish anything. Eventually, of course, you realize there are limits. But you learn medicine with the sense that you'll be able to take control of the body, manage it, turn the troubled ship around.

As a young doctor, you learn all the theory. You do the training. Before I started my internship, I had to do an advanced cardiac life support training through the American Heart Association. With all the training, you think it's going to work just like during your practice runs. When you do your practice runs, of course, they want to make you feel good about it. You get a rhythm. The patient survives and walks out. In reality, that doesn't happen as often as we like—in fact, in a majority of cases it doesn't happen.

When you realize that, two main things can happen. You either feel very humbled, or you respond by exerting more control. The whole idea of autonomy and control is really one of the main tenets for euthanasia: if you can't fix it, then kill it. From a purely medical perspective, it is so wrong because, in a very large sense, there's never a point when you can truly say, "There's nothing more to do."

"Nothing more to do" can range from meaning achieving a one hundred percent cure to "we won't be able to turn this disease around" to "maybe we can at least slow it down." Even if you can just slow it down, there is something more to do. Maybe that something is just making a patient's life more comfortable. That doesn't mean you've done nothing. On the contrary, you've improved something.

If the person can have a few more days, that's something. It can give time to say goodbye to somebody who needs that closure. I've worked in intensive care units where a nurse will say, "There's nothing more to do. You can just disconnect the ventilator with the family's permission."

And I'll answer, "Well, let's talk to the family. Let's see what they want to do, get them involved."

In a code room where people who have undergone a cardiac arrest are being resuscitated, after twenty minutes[6] there might be very little chance of turning things around so, again, a nurse will say, "There's nothing more to do. Maybe we should just stop it."

My response is always, "Let's continue until we speak to the family so they can have time to be involved in that decision and know what the situation is."

[6] This is the amount of time recommended by the American Heart Association 2010 guidelines, taking into account multiple factors including age, underlying health status, delay in initiating CPR, whether the arrest was witnessed, and whether the heart was defibrillated. However, some studies indicate that even longer times can be associated with good outcomes. The 2015 guidelines do not provide a time limit because of insufficient data (American Heart Association, *2015 AHA Guidelines Update for CPR and ECC*, available at https://www.cercp.org/images/stories/recursos/Guias%202015/Guidelines-RCP-AHA-2015-Full.pdf).

A recent study states, "There is generally a better neurological outcome with a shorter duration of CPR in survivors of cardiac arrest, However a cut-off beyond which resuscitation is likely to lead to unfavourable outcome was not possible to determine and is unlikely to exist, as many people survive prolonged cardiac arrest with minimal consequences. There is not enough evidence to create a definitive rule for termination of CPR in the hospital setting. Clinicians should continue to take into account that in many cases the chance of neurologically favourable survival decreases the longer CPR is continued, however this alone is not enough to make the decision to terminate efforts." (Clare Welbourn & Nikolaos Efstathiou, (2018), "How Does the Length of Cardiopulmonary Resuscitation Affect Brain Damage in Patients Surviving Cardiac Arrest? A Systematic Review," *Scandinavian Journal of Trauma, Resuscitation and Emergency Medicine* 26, no. 77 (2018)).

Finally, Matos et. al. argue that for children, performing CPR for more than twenty minutes and even beyond thirty-five minutes was not futile in some patient illness categories, especially those undergoing cardiac surgery (Renée I. Matos, R. Scott Watson, Vinay M. Nadkarni, Hsin-Hui Huang, et. al., "Duration of Cardiopulmonary Resuscitation and Illness Category Impact Survival and Neurologic Outcomes for In-hospital Pediatric Cardiac Arrests," *Circulation* 127, no. 4 (2013)).

I think it is far better to allow the family to be there, knowing that you've made the effort and that you still care, rather than just stopping and walking out. You need to tell them clearly so they know you have done everything. They see the effort that's been made. Of course, for some people, watching someone being resuscitated is a very scary thing and they don't want to see it. But they need to be asked if they would like to be there. They need to know we're still trying, or even that we're planning to stop once we've gone as far as we can.

Bringing the family into the situation, into the decision making, can seem to some like giving up medical control. But giving up control, in that sense, can become a very positive thing. When you use it as justification for saying, "We're going to inject somebody because there's nothing more to do," you lose the crucial importance of seeing life come and go. You reduce life and death to a mechanical medical routine. You risk forgetting that while every life must end, we are all made to live.

My unshakeable conviction about that, which drove me to join with the Physicians' Alliance against Euthanasia[7] battling Medical Aid in Dying in Canada, and to launch costly legal challenges against the legislation, comes not only from my experience as a physician and from my personal Christian convictions, but also from my own remembrance of death, near-death, and life that was renewed when it seemed there was nothing more to do.

The earliest memory I have of death was my grandfather's. I was four years old and boarding a plane to fly to the west coast of the United States. I remember getting up at three in the morning so we could catch the plane—a DC-3—through Chicago. The trip became a family story my mom told later—we'd missed a connection, and the airlines had put the five of us up in a hotel as we were heading to the funeral.

---

[7] See https://collectifmedecins.org/en/.

He was my mom's dad, a plaster and cement contractor, who died suddenly at sixty-seven. I never really knew my grandparents, but having that story about going to his funeral, being able to pass it and other family stories along to my children, has been very important for me. His death and his funeral when I was a child are my connection to his life.

My own father, John, died in his late seventies after developing diabetes and suffering a fractured pelvis in a fall. Caring for him through his illness motivated me to ensure that those who were seriously ill would receive the best of care. It inspired me to found the Coalition of Physicians for Social Justice in Montreal, Canada. But the true inspiration was this man's life—this man who lived until his natural death, this man who was born in the same five-family building where I grew up in Lachine.

Our home was a small dwelling with two bedrooms housing a family of six. I used to sleep on the sofa when I was a child until we purchased bunk beds. An aunt and uncle lived next door.

My dad worked tirelessly to provide for the family. He started his career in the grocery business, but Mom insisted that he not sell cigarettes and beer in his little grocery store. She said that it would ruin the health and lives of our neighbours. Since small grocers were expected to stock those items, my dad gave up the store and joined his brother Charles in the clothing business.

My dad was always generous with whatever he had. During the Second World War, many fathers from Italian families were interned in camps. There was a fear they might be Mussolini sympathizers. My dad would give mittens and socks to the fire chief, who collected items for the impoverished Italian children being raised alone by their moms.

As his health declined, my dad was often left alone in the hospital with little attention to his basic needs. We spent a lot of time at his bedside. We hired private help to make sure his healthcare needs were met. It was a painful time for me and for my family to see his condition grow worse. What mattered above all was that we, as a family, could stay with him until his last breath.

To the extent his life inspired me, so too did his death. I realized that many seniors were not always getting the best nutritional support in hospitals. As a result, I helped organize conferences to raise awareness of the need for better nutrition of seniors. We educated hundreds of dietitians, doctors, nurses, and healthcare workers.

Would a Medical Aid in Dying injection, had it been legally available, created a simpler, easier routine for all of us? Maybe. But think what would have been lost by opting for the medically mechanical, the healthcare routine. I, as a doctor, wouldn't have learned so much that I needed to know and would end up passing on to others. We, as a family, wouldn't have been there to give back to him all that he had given to us, and to so many. Most importantly of all, for us as Christians, we wouldn't have answered our God-given call to charity—that is, to love with the sacrificial love that Jesus Christ gives us.

At a purely practical, secular level we might also have thrown in the towel too soon by saying "there's nothing more that can be done" while hope still remained alive. That represents a human and spiritual misdiagnosis that poses disastrous risks, as I've seen with my own eyes.

In the case of my father-in-law Tony, I believe it would have been tantamount to murder. Tony was essentially given up for dead in 2010. Years later, he's still very much alive and vital.

My wife's father collapsed in the emergency room in Italy when he was on vacation. He was operated on originally for appendicitis, but when they did the pathology, they detected signet cell cancer, which is a very aggressive form. It's one of the worst intestinal cancers you can get.

He came back to Montreal, where he was operated on by an amazing team at our community hospital. Still, things went from bad to worse. He had to undergo multiple surgeries, his bowels were leaking, and he ended up in intensive care. He was in so much pain that they couldn't alleviate it while he was conscious, so they had to put him into what we call palliative sedation and intubate him.

It was a form of palliative care. Everyone said there was no chance of him coming through bowel infection and organ failure. But eventually, through amazing medical care and what some people would call a miracle, things turned around. Sometimes we pray for people and things don't improve. In this case, they did.

We've since traveled to Italy together. Tony still works in the garage he started and that his son has taken over. He does Italian gardening every summer. He grows fig trees, which he puts into the ground and brings up every spring. You have to be in pretty good shape to do that.

I wasn't able to know my grandparents, but I did everything to ensure that the only grandfather my children have could make it through. There were no guarantees. To me, that is really the whole issue of life and death. We can't guarantee outcomes; we can't guarantee that people won't die. But I strongly believe each of us has a time to live. We aren't to diminish that time. I share that belief with my patients. I tell them, "This may be your time, but we will never know unless we try," which is not a fatalistic attitude. Fatalism for me is giving up before even trying because we believe that no matter what we do, it won't make a difference. But what we do *does* make a difference, even if it isn't what we had hoped for. It can be as simple as touching someone's life by our efforts and caring.

I believe what the Bible says: there's a time and season for everything, and with God, the years are numbered for each person.

But it's not for us to number them. It's not for us to cut them short. It's for us to do our best to give people the largest number. If we succeed, that's wonderful, and if we don't, it's not because we didn't try.

Consider someone who is faced with a very terrible future and decides to end their life. For me, that is equivalent to euthanasia and assisted suicide. Yet in such a situation, we do everything to try to stop people from killing themselves. We provide people with hope. We help them to understand there's always something to live for. In the same way, if a person wants to end their life because of a terminal disease, our obligation is to tell that person, "You know what? We're still going to be there for you. We're not going to abandon you."

I deal with people with severe neurological diseases such as Lou Gehrig's. One woman I treated lived and saw her grandchildren. Ultimately her physician had to turn off the ventilator, but she persisted right to the end and did not suffer. We didn't abandon her, because to abandon her would be to abandon hope. Hope guides us to live until the natural end, but it is also there to drive us to cure many of these diseases. It's working out our God-given capacity to cure many diseases that we were unable to cure in the past.

Christ healed lepers and ordered us to follow His example and heal the sick. He did it by miracles, but we can do it with our scientific knowledge and our technological ability. What's lacking is will. We can do so much more. I've worked in the developing world and seen projects that Canada and the United States were involved in that made me very proud. Let's do more. Let's develop cures for Lou Gehrig's, for Parkinson's, for dementia, for children's diseases in the developing world.

Let's not do less. Let's not accept death as routine, prematurely saying, "There's nothing more we can do." When that's done under the pretext of Medical Aid in Dying, we're treating that patient like a body, not a person. We're forgetting that person has a human story for which he or she was made to live.

Chapter 4

MAID MYTHS AND REALITY CHECKS

One of the arguments used in favour of assisted suicide compares it with informed consent for surgery. The argument is put forward that when a patient gives informed consent for surgery, they don't know the outcome. Something might go wrong. They might die. Informed consent by its nature accepts death as a potential outcome weighed against the patient's willingness to take the risk.

The fallacy, of course, is that with assisted suicide or euthanasia, death is not a risk—it's a certainty. With surgery, or even taking medication, there's no iron-clad guarantee you won't have a severe reaction even though everything possible is done to avoid that. However, with euthanasia or assisted suicide, it's a one hundred percent guarantee that you're not coming through it.

Yet there's a significant percentage of people who do give informed consent to euthanasia or assisted suicide, and then withdraw their consent before (obviously) the injection is administered. One report shows it's as high as twenty percent.[8] If people who've

---

[8] In a Quebec review of 377 non-administered euthanasia deaths, seventy-nine people had changed their minds about wanting to die. (Gaétan Barrette, Minister of Health and Social Services, "Commission sur les Soins de Fin de Vie: Rapport Annuel d'Activités, 1er Juillet 2016–30 Juin 2017." Report submitted to National Assembly of Quebec. Available at http://www.assnat.qc.ca/fr/travaux-parlementaires/assemblee-nationale/41-1/journal-debats/20171026so/documents-deposes.html.)

consented to final injections had more time, would even more withdraw? What if they spoke to a psychologist? Or met a new doctor? What if something unforeseen changed in their family or social circumstances?

Did those who changed their minds have better pain control? Did they receive more love and support? Was there some other change in their life? Was there a better outlook? The study didn't look at these questions.

A media story here in Montreal tells of a patient who wanted to die until a neighbour came over and made him some soup. He changed his mind about giving up and wanting to die. So many factors can change. Informed consent, then, means a willingness to take a calculated risk for life. It can never be consent to be put to death. Death may ensue because of a refusal of treatment or withdrawal of treatment, but this isn't a guarantee. Neither is this the same as intentionally provoking death by a lethal injection.

When it's surgery or pharmaceuticals, the person doing the informing has a body of knowledge about what the probabilities are. They know the desired outcome, and they know what the contraindications are. But when it comes to death, they don't know any more than anybody else. They know the person's dead, but they don't know what that actually means. None of us do.

Advocates for euthanasia and assisted suicide will say, "Yes, but we allow patients to change their mind right up to the end." But when they've stopped breathing because you've paralyzed their lungs, how can they express what's on their mind? And you as the doctor, the nurse, the healthcare professional, certainly can't read their mind. Once the procedure begins, there's no changing anyone's mind. It's magical thinking to believe otherwise.

Yet the myth of informed consent has been an important part of driving Canada into a full-on embrace of euthanasia and assisted suicide. I came up against it in my court battle to stop the legislation being put into effect in Quebec.

It is far from the only myth that's been employed. I once tried to list all the myths I've encountered since finding myself in the battle against so-called Medical Aid in Dying. I stopped once I got past one hundred. I want to deal in this chapter with five that I believe are critical to return us to realistic—not magical or mythical—thinking about what's at stake.

Here are those five myths, and their corresponding reality checks:

MYTH 1. Classifying euthanasia and assisted suicide as "medical treatment" automatically makes them acceptable and therefore "safe" when administered by a doctor or healthcare professional.

The *reality* is that deliberately taking a human life remains killing regardless of who commits it. A doctor who kills may be doing so in his or her professional capacity. But he or she has still intentionally killed. The key word is *intentional*. Killing requires intention, which is what distinguishes it from dying. We will all die. Until the advent of euthanasia and assisted suicide, only a small minority of us—soldiers, police officers or victims of violent crime—were ever in real and present danger of being killed.

The appeal of putting killing in the hands of healthcare professionals to make it safe runs into the reality, then, of what I've noted in earlier chapters about medicine being a fallible profession prone to mechanical routine and path of least resistance solutions. But it also runs into the even deeper reality exemplified by a woman I know named Jeannette.

Jeannette is an elegant, retired woman who worked for many years in my dad's clothing store. She called me one day in 2012 in great distress. Although I was not her family doctor, she wanted clarification and encouragement. She had been told that she had lung cancer. She was, of course, devastated. The diagnosis was confirmed by her lung specialist after multiple scans. She shared with me that, prior to undergoing surgery, she went to the famous St. Joseph's Oratory in Montreal to pray and ask for divine intervention. She told me that before her surgery she was confident that she did not have lung cancer and told her surgeon the same. She then underwent a partial removal of her lung. After several weeks of anxious waiting, she was given the pathology results. To the surprise of all her physicians, she did not have lung cancer.

Did her prayer result in a miracle cure for Jeannette? Are other medical explanations probable? The answer to such questions is an emphatic "We just don't know for sure."

But Jeannette believes—and I agree with her—that there is one thing we can know: if euthanasia or assisted suicide had been available in 2012, some people in her situation would jump for it, fearing the worst—even if the diagnosis was wrong; even if a remission, a cure, a miracle remained possible.

That risk is why the myth of making euthanasia and assisted suicide "safe" by making it "medical" must be debunked. Far from it being safe, there is a very real danger in putting euthanasia or assisted suicide in the same light as medical care. A wrong diagnosis, a loss of hope, or a very human desire to take the path of least resistance, could all short-circuit someone's life by inducing them to plunge headlong into assisted suicide or euthanasia.

There is nothing safe about such a prospect, regardless of how well-trained, competent, or credentialled those who administer medical killing might be.

MYTH 2. Canada is an advanced progressive society where the social and healthcare needs of its citizens are fully met. Euthanasia or assisted suicide is a personal choice that must be open to those suffering and wanting to die.

The *reality* is that Canada has inadequate healthcare services for many of its citizens.[9] Many people do not have their basic needs met, including affordable housing and nutrition. They want to live in dignity, rather than die by euthanasia or assisted suicide. The ill-effects of that inadequacy are embodied in the circumstances of Lisa D'Amico, who lives with cerebral palsy. When I first met Lisa, I was touched by her bravery. She struggles daily, living life one day at a time. Every step is painful as she drags herself with a walker. She can afford to eat only one or two meals a day.

She needs physical therapy and hydrotherapy to relieve her pain. Neither of these services are covered by the Canadian public healthcare system outside the hospital, and she cannot afford to pay for these services.

She has publicly declared that the government wants to "force her to accept euthanasia" by depriving her and people like her of basic services and supports that would make her life bearable. Her purpose in life is not to die in dignity: she wants to *live* in dignity. She wants care and support. As CTV News has reported,

> D'Amico said she is hopeless, that her life is not going anywhere, and the lack of care makes her feel worthless.

---

[9] According a Commonwealth Fund report published in 2017, Canada is ranked third from last for healthcare systems among eleven developed countries (Monique Scotti, "Canada's Health-Care System is Third-Last in New Ranking of Developed Countries," *Global News*, July 14, 2017 (https://globalnews.ca/news/3599458/canadas-health-care-system-lower-performing-compared-to-its-peers-study/)).

"I want to be free. I don't want to die," said D'Amico, but added that life was difficult without access to proper care, proper food, and proper technical aid to alleviate her disability.

"If I ever require euthanasia, it's not my disability that's killing me, it's my own government." [10]

The reality of death being prescribed for lack of resources was reported in a local Quebec newspaper on November 30, 2019. Raymond, a nursing home resident with a neurological condition, was going to be euthanized because his living conditions had become intolerable: the lack of air conditioning in the summer and the lack of privacy.[11]

The systemic failure to provide for people like Raymond and Lisa adequately is what makes the myth of euthanasia and assisted suicide as personal choice so pernicious. There is grievous danger in making so-called MAiD not only acceptable but a solution for resource-strapped healthcare systems. As a doctor, I regularly attend meetings where cost-management of patient care is discussed frankly between physicians, nurses, and hospital administrators. They argue that they are forced to ration the public healthcare dollars spent on patient care because of the budgetary envelope.

I hear it all the time: "We have only so much money. We have to set a limit." But if we comply, we may not end up doing all the necessary investigations to find the best treatment for the patient. It's already there. Patients and families are encouraged to downgrade the level of care. Physicians are afraid that their

---

[10] Vanessa Lee & Solarina Ho, "Two Canadians Want Next Prime Minister to Push for 'Assisted Living,' Not Assisted Dying," *CTV News,* Oct. 1, 2019 (https://www.ctvnews.ca/health/two-canadians-want-next-prime-minister-to-push-for-assistance-in-living-not-assisted-dying-1.4619767).

[11] Mélanie Noël, "Dénoncer avant de mourir," *La Tribune,* November 30, 2019 (https://www.latribune.ca/actualites/denoncer-avant-de-mourir-video-6b5b5b9901c42d9660ec5ba19a0eda78).

hospital privileges could be withdrawn if they "cross the line" of over-utilizing resources that benefit the patient but are considered too costly. These physicians could be considered "out of the norm," and thus an overly conscientious physician may appear to be "problematic."

With the best of intentions, medical healthcare workers including doctors and nurses pre-occupied about hospital spending can influence individuals to abruptly end their life through MAiD. Moreover, under the guise of "co-management," they may resort to suggesting the least costly treatments: euthanasia or assisted suicide. Simply raising the possibility of a patient ending their life through euthanasia or assisted suicide has a major influence in encouraging patients to a hastened death. As noted by Barbara Kay,

> Physicians greatly influence their decision-making. In a 2001 interview Dutch physician Joke Groen-Evers noted that, when talking with a terminal patient, she would feel bound to bring up the subject of euthanasia: "And nine times out of ten the patient would return with a request for euthanasia." Finding herself more comfortable suggesting palliative care, she stopped using the "E-word." "And what do you know: almost no one asks for it anymore! … If you mention euthanasia, they will ask for it. If you mention palliative care, then that is what they will choose."[12]

Euthanasia or assisted suicide are the least costly alternatives for cost-conscious administrators. The cost savings has been confirmed, and it is publicized to physicians in a January 2017 article of the *Canadian Medical Association Journal*,

---

[12] Barbara Kay, "No One Really Wants Euthanasia. Suffering People Want an End to Their Pain," *National Post*, February 4, 2015.

"Cost Analysis of Medical Assistance in Dying in Canada." It concludes: "Providing medical assistance in dying in Canada should not result in any excess financial burden to the health-care system, and could result in substantial savings."[13]

With people like Lisa D'Amico having to choose between food and care even in Canada, and the inexorable pressures healthcare professionals and administrators alike are under to meet budgets, it is irresponsible to perpetuate the myth that euthanasia and assisted suicide are never the result of severe external pressures, and that they are pure rational choices freely arrived at by citizens of a civilized and caring country. On the contrary, *the reality is that both the medical system, coupled with a lack of proper social service care, can manipulate Canadians into choosing premature death.*

MYTH 3. Euthanasia or assisted suicide is just a next step in palliative care.

The ***reality*** is that intentional ending of life is the exact opposite of palliative care. It is being used as a de facto alternative to palliative care. Why? Because there is such a shortage of palliative care in Canada. The majority of Canadians don't have access to it—either at home or in long-term facilities. In long-term facilities where residents have less than six months to live, only one in five receive palliative care, while only fifteen percent of people who die at home receive palliative care.[14]

A case from my own practice demonstrates what a gamble getting proper palliative care remains in this country after years of

---

[13] Aaron J. Trachtenberg & Braden Manns, "Cost Analysis of Medical Assistance in Dying in Canada," *Canadian Medical Association Journal* 189, no. 3 (2017): E101–E105.

[14] Canadian Institute for Health Information, *Access to Palliative Care in Canada* (Ottawa, ON: CIHI, 2018) (https://www.cihi.ca/sites/default/files/document/access-palliative-care-2018-en-web.pdf).

promises from the federal and provincial government to improve its availability and access.

Judith has been my patient for many years. She shared with me the story of her mother, who died peaceably of liver cancer in a private palliative care facility in Montreal in January 2015. In stark contrast, her close friend's dad suffered at home in the last months of his life because of the lack of access to palliative care.

Judith's story isn't just another bit of unsubstantiated anecdotal evidence. The Quebec College of Physicians, which is mandated to ensure the quality of medical practice, issued a letter signed by their director, Charles Bernard, to the Quebec government on May 29, 2018 expressing their concerns that physician-assisted death might be causing patients to turn to lethal injections because of the lack of palliative care.

In clear language, the College informed the health minister about "difficulties with the accessibility of palliative care for many end-of-life patients" and warned that "in certain well-identified cases, some patients, not benefiting from such care, could have had no choice but to request medical assistance in dying to end their days 'in dignity.'" The College of Physicians firmly reminded the minister that "end-of-life care cannot be limited to access to medical assistance in dying."[15] As Dr. Bernard argued, "provincial foot-dragging on plans to substantially expand palliative care services is actually denying patients the very choice that was promised in the shift to MAiD, and making it increasingly problematic to discern which patients truly wanted to have a doctor deliberately end their life."[16]

---

[15] *Collège des Médecins du Québec*, "Objet: *Accès à des soins palliatifs de qualité* au *Québec*," May 29, 2018. Letter to Dr. Gaetan Barrette, legally acquired through access of information. Translated by Dr. Paul Saba.

[16] Peter Stockland, "Assisted Dying Was Supposed to Be an Option. To Some Patients, It Looks Like the Only One," *Macleans*, June 22, 2018 (https://www.macleans.ca/society/assisted-dying-was-supposed-to-be-an-option-to-some-patients-it-looks-like-the-only-one/).

The very need for Quebec's chief governing body for quality of medicine to send and publicize a letter containing such graphic warnings shows how deep the confusion between euthanasia/assisted suicide and palliative care has become. It is crucial we restore the reality that they are not the same thing in any way. The difference is made crystal clear by the World Health Organization's Definition of Palliative Care: [17]

> Palliative care is an approach that improves the quality of life of patients and their families facing the problem associated with life-threatening illness, through the prevention and relief of suffering by means of early identification and impeccable assessment and treatment of pain and other problems, physical, psychosocial and spiritual.

According to the WHO, palliative care:[18]

- provides relief from pain and other distressing symptoms;
- affirms life and regards dying as a normal process;
- intends neither to hasten or postpone death;
- integrates the psychological and spiritual aspects of patient care;
- offers a support system to help patients live as actively as possible until death;
- offers a support system to help the family cope during the patient's illness and in their own bereavement;
- uses a team approach to address the needs of patients and their families, including bereavement counselling, if indicated;

---

[17] WHO Definition of Palliative Care, *World Health Organization* (https://www.who.int/cancer/palliative/definition/en/).
[18] Ibid.

- will enhance quality of life, and may also positively influence the course of illness;
- is applicable early in the course of illness, in conjunction with other therapies that are intended to prolong life, such as chemotherapy or radiation therapy, and includes those investigations needed to better understand and manage distressing clinical complications.

The difference between those characteristics and injecting a patient with a toxic substance to stop their breathing and, ultimately, their heart, could not be more pronounced. Again, intentionality is the key word. The intention of palliative care is to relieve suffering. The intention of euthanasia and assisted suicide is to eliminate the sufferer. Medical literature shows how effectively good palliative care can achieve its goal.

A classic study in the *New England Journal of Medicine* compared patients with metastatic non-small cell lung cancer who received early palliative care along with standard oncologic care to those who received cancer treatment without palliative care. Those who received palliative care had better quality of life with less depression, and longer median survival of almost three months.[19]

In a study conducted by Dartmouth Medical School in New Hampshire, patients receiving palliative care along with oncology care had higher scores for quality of life than those receiving usual oncology care alone.

Patients with advanced heart or lung disease or cancer, with a life expectancy between one to five years, found palliative care acceptable and helpful, reported increased satisfaction and

---

[19] Jennifer S. Temel, Joseph A. Greer, Alona Muzikansky, et al., "Early Palliative Care for Patients with Metastatic Non-Small-Cell Lung Cancer," New England Journal of Medicine 363 (2010): 733.

decreased healthcare utilization, and were more likely to die at home.[20]

People who receive quality palliative care report less suffering, better quality of life, and improved survival. People who receive palliative care early on live happier and longer lives. People who receive euthanasia or assisted suicide end up dead. That is the blunt reason why euthanasia and assisted suicide are not part, and must never be, part of palliative care.

A grim reality in Canada and Quebec, however, is that a lack of palliative care services is pushing some people to seek euthanasia or assisted suicide out of desperation. For most people needing palliative care, choice is an illusion.

MYTH 4. Euthanasia or assisted suicide will always be limited to only a small number of exceptional cases. Anyone who disagrees is indulging in a slippery slope argument.

Real facts to counter this myth have long been available directly from Belgium. In that small country, in ***reality*** there was a sizable increase in the number of euthanasia deaths in the first twelve years after legalization. In 2003, there were 235 euthanasia deaths. There were 2,021 deaths by 2015, representing an increase of 760 percent. That's in a population base of about eleven million, one-third of Canada's. Nearby in the Netherlands, the number of official cases of euthanasia rose from the official report of 1,815 in 2003[21] to 6,091 in 2016. It's a 235 percent increase. On a population

[20] M.W. Rabow, K. Schanche, J. Petersen, et al., "Patient Perceptions of an Outpatient Palliative Care Intervention: 'It Had Been on my Mind Before, but I Did Not Know How to Start Talking about Death…'" *Journal of Pain Symptom Management* 26, no. 5 (2003): 1010.

[21] Alex Schadenburg, "Sharp Growth in Dutch Euthanasia Deaths," *Euthanasia Prevention Coalition* (blog), June 16, 2010, http://alexschadenberg.blogspot.com/2010/06/sharp-growth-in-dutch-euthanasia-deaths.html.

base of about seventeen million, euthanasia now accounts for four percent of total deaths[22] in the Netherlands.

A study published in the British Medical Journal[23] reviewed one hundred Belgian patients who had a psychiatric diagnosis and requested euthanasia between October 2007 and December 2011. The patients included the depressed and those with personality disorders or autism. None had life-threatening or life-ending illness. In this group, thirty-five euthanasia deaths were carried out.

According to another study published in the British Medical Journal,[24] forty-two people in the Netherlands were euthanized for a psychiatric disorder without any life-ending physical illness. The majority of these people were depressed.

It is noteworthy that Belgium extended euthanasia to children on February 13, 2014, just as Quebec was on the verge of legalizing euthanasia. Despite those ominous and abundantly reported warning signs, Quebec's minister of health declared at the time of announcement of the province's "historic" bill to legalize euthanasia that "probably none, or a handful of people" would request it.[25] Between June 2016 and June 2017, 634 people were euthanized in Quebec,[26] triple the number in Belgium when its experiment with euthanasia first began.

[22] "Number of Official Cases of Euthanasia Rises 10% in the Netherlands," *DutchNews.nl,* April 12, 2017, https://www.dutchnews.nl/news/2017/04/number-of-official-cases-of-euthanasia-rise-10-in-the-netherlands/.

[23] Lieve Thienpont, Monica Verhofstadt, Tony Van Loon, et al., "Euthanasia Requests, Procedures and Outcomes for 100 Belgian Patients Suffering from Psychiatric Disorders: A Retrospective, Descriptive Study," *BMJ Open* 5:e007454. doi: 10.1136/bmjopen-2014-007454.

[24] Udo Schuklenk & Suzanne van de Vathorst, "Treatment-Resistant Major Depressive Disorder and Assisted Dying," *Journal of Medical Ethics* 41 (2015): 577-583.

[25] Grame Hamilton, "'We're Not Expecting Hordes of Patients': Quebec Health Minister on Historic Bill to Legalize Euthanasia," *National Post*, December 2, 2015.

[26] Gaétan Barrette, Minister of Health and Social Services, "Commission sur les Soins de Fin de Vie: Rapport Annuel d'Activités, 1er Juillet 2016–30 Juin 2017." Report submitted to National Assembly of Quebec. Available at http://www.assnat.qc.ca/fr/travaux-parlementaires/assemblee-nationale/41-1/journal-debats/20171026so/documents-deposes.html.

Projections are always tricky, of course, but Rabbi Raphael Afilalo, a director of pastoral services at the Jewish General Hospital in Montreal, estimates that more than 2.4 million people globally will die this way every year—and he is taking into account only the world's fifty most populous countries. His calculation[27] uses the ratio of .038 percent of the total population, or 6,386 annual deaths, to Holland's population of 16.8 million. However the numbers are extrapolated, that is an extremely large "handful" of people having their natural lives cut short by toxic injection.

Yet there is an even more frightful reality than just the raw numbers. It is the seemingly inexorable expansion of euthanasia and assisted suicide to deal with an increasingly wider range of illnesses and kinds of suffering. The reason is that once medicine is used to kill, new norms are constantly emerging. The mindset of society will shift to accommodate things that were unthinkable only a short time before.

In Belgium, the legislation initially specified the practice of euthanasia for adults who were suffering unbearably and "terminally ill." Despite this, and beyond euthanasia being extended to children, it is now being debated for those who are "tired of life," for the depressed, and for those who do not believe their quality of life is worth living.[28]

Case reports in the media have exposed the euthanasia stories of an anorexic woman in her forties, deaf twins in their forties who feared going blind, a man in his forties who wasn't happy with his sex change operation, and a grandmother who was euthanized

---

[27] Janice Arnold, "Assisted Death Forbidden, Rabbi Tells Ethics Conference," *The Canadian Jewish News,* June 15, 2015 (https://www.cjnews.com/news/canada/assisted-death-forbidden-rabbi-tells-ethics-conference).

[28] Raphael Cohen-Almagor, "Euthanizing People Who Are 'Tired of Life' in Belgium," in *Euthanasia and Assisted Suicide: Lessons from Belgium,* David Albert Jones, Chris Gastmans & Calum MacKellar, eds. (Cambridge: Cambridge University Press, 2017), 188–201.

for depression, leaving behind grieving children and very young grandchildren.

Here in Canada, on April 1, 2018—less than two years after the legalization of Medical Aid in Dying—it was reported that a couple married for seventy-three years were euthanized together. The husband, who had health issues including "fainting," "heart-related problems," and "age-related frailty," didn't want to be left alone after his wife decided to have her life ended prematurely because of chronic health conditions including rheumatoid arthritis. Neither husband nor wife was actively dying. They were well enough to spend a romantic dinner evening together at their favorite restaurant.[29]

In Ontario, the Provincial-Territorial Expert Advisory Group on Physician-Assisted Dying is recommending euthanasia without parental consent for children as young as eleven years old. Recommendation 17 contends that, "Access to physician-assisted dying should not be impeded by the imposition of arbitrary age limits. Provinces and territories should recommend that the federal government make it clear in its changes to the Criminal Code that eligibility for physician-assisted dying is to be based on competence rather than age."[30]

Amid all the reports and statistics, however, it is the direct experience of a patient of mine that both confirms and illustrates how the medical death mindset expands, and how it pushes us to forget that we were made to live. The case of Sylvain and his wife Sherley resolved very happily. For how many others in similar circumstances, though, might it have ended tragically?

---

[29] Kelly Grant, "Medically Assisted Death Allows Couple Married Almost 73 Years to Die Together," *Globe and Mail,* April 1, 2018.

[30] Provincial-Territorial Expert Advisory Group on Physician-Assisted Dying, "Final Report," Nov. 30, 2015 (http://www.health.gov.on.ca/en/news/bulletin/2015/docs/eagreport_20151214_en.pdf).

Sylvain and Sherley have a young daughter, Jolyanne. Before Jolyanne was born, a routine ultrasound demonstrated severe anomalies, including Down syndrome, and a defective esophagus. They were offered abortion to avoid birthing a severely handicapped child with little chance of survival. They said "no." As with my own daughter, Jessica, the decision was made as a family to allow the pregnancy to continue to its natural conclusion. Against all odds, and after multiple surgeries, Jolyanne survived. Like Jessica, she did not have Down's.

A few years later, I received a call from Sylvain one evening at my office. He was crying and obviously in great emotional distress. Sherley, only in her forties, was in a coma and on life support. The physicians were advising him to pull the plug. He was told that after twenty days on life support, there was "little chance" his wife would recover to a "reasonable quality of life."

Sherley was on ventilator life support because of severe lung pneumonia in the context of a reduced immune system from bone cancer. I advised Sylvain to come to my office to talk the next day. After a long discussion, he asked me to call the treating physician at the hospital. Sylvain wanted everything possible done to save his wife. He refused to take her off life support.

Because her care required more than the local hospital could offer, Sherley was transferred to the Montreal General Hospital. She later walked out of the hospital. Sylvain says he would be alone today without the two women he loves most in his life if he had believed his doctors' predictions and followed their advice.

I have no doubt the doctors involved sincerely believed they were giving that advice in the absolute best interests of the patients. They would have no trouble convincing anyone that their advice demonstrated complete medical competence and respect for prevailing medical ethics.

Yet it also demonstrates how the medical administration of death expands to cover the number of conditions available to it. In earlier chapters, I referred to the routine mechanization of medicine. When it becomes the healthcare norm, the patient becomes a problem to be solved. Death becomes the obvious and ever ready solution. *In such circumstances, it is obvious that assisted suicide and euthanasia will expand exponentially as the categories are nonchalantly broadened.*

MYTH 5. We lose our meaning as human beings unless we are young, successful, in full health, and enjoying the best "quality of life" possible.

Nadine[31] is a young woman whose **reality** utterly refutes this myth that lies at the heart of euthanasia and assisted suicide. At the age of fourteen, Nadine suffered unbelievably. She underwent multiple rounds of chemotherapy, and a failed bone marrow transplant that almost cost her life. She was told that she had little chance to survive. There were times when she wanted only to die.

The head of the World Federation of Right to Die Societies has said it would be a good thing for euthanasia to be available to young people in the situation Nadine faced.[32]

"They're nauseated. They don't want to go through with the third or fourth chemotherapy. They say, 'I just want to stop, this is no life for me anymore," Rob Jonquiere, an architect of the Netherlands euthanasia law, is quoted in media reports.[33]

Yet because Nadine couldn't give up, she didn't. Euthanasia and euthanasia doctors weren't available to inject Nadine when she was going through her battle against leukemia.

---

[31] "SOS … Les Québécois Lancent un Cri du Cœur pour STOPPER l'Euthanasie," *Newswire*, Feb. 9, 2014 (https://www.newswire.ca/news-releases/sos--les-quebecois-lancent-un-cri-du-cur-pour-stopper-leuthanasie-513699571.html).

[32] Sharon Kirkey, "Proposal to Extend Euthanasia to Children 'Is Very Dangerous,' Top Medical Ethicist Says," *National Post*, December 15, 2015.

[33] Ibid.

Instead, she was surrounded by the loving support of her sister and mother. Today she is a young woman in her twenties, having completed college with a hopeful attitude toward the future. If she had been immersed in the mythology of euthanasia and assisted suicide, she would have lacked that hope. Her life would have seemed meaningless. Her life would have been lost.

Long before Nadine, one of the twentieth century's most eminent doctors discovered just how powerful a force hope and meaning can be in human life. Viktor Frankl was an eminent Austrian neurologist and psychiatrist. He also survived the Nazi death camps of the Second World War. Out of that experience, he wrote one of the great inspirational books, rooted in practical observation of behaviour, called *Man's Search for Meaning*.

A central assertion of the book is Frankl's first-hand observation, through the eyes of someone with a doctorate in medicine, that the individuals who survived the slave labour, the hunger, the cold, the degradation, and the suffering of the Holocaust, though they varied in many ways, were those who would not waver from the conviction that we are made to live. In fact, Frankl identifies key signs he noted in those who were about to die. One of the most crucial was a loss of meaning. Immediately following it was a loss of hope.

"Those who have a 'why' to live, can bear with almost any 'how,'" Frankl writes in *Man's Search for Meaning*, quoting Nietzsche.[34] "In some ways suffering ceases to be suffering at the moment it finds a meaning, such as the meaning of a sacrifice."[35] He also understands that love is the ultimate source of meaning. "The salvation of man is through love and in love."[36]

In Nadine's case, as in the others I've cited so far in this book,

[34] Available at https://www.goodreads.com/quotes/137-he-who-has-a-why-to-live-for-can-bear.

[35] Available at https://www.goodreads.com/quotes/55188-in-some-ways-suffering-ceases-to-be-suffering-at-the.

[36] Available at https://www.goodreads.com/quotes/958322-the-salvation-of-man-is-

the moment of meaning arrived with the awareness of being surrounded by those who loved them, cared for them, and would be with them through recovery or until the end, whichever life had in store. To have been killed prematurely would have extinguished any possibility of that moment flowering.

Euthanasia and assisted suicide throw away the lives of people who might otherwise have many happy years to live. But they even discard the precious seconds that would have otherwise been available for love to flourish.

We must never forget that our lives are valuable in themselves because they are gifts of hope, of meaning, and especially of love. We must always remember the corollary: love doesn't care about our age, our wealth, our infirmities, our quality of life. Love tells us we have meaning regardless of anything of those things. *The reality of love is all the proof we need that we are made to live, and we are made to love and be loved.*

---

through-love-and-in-love.

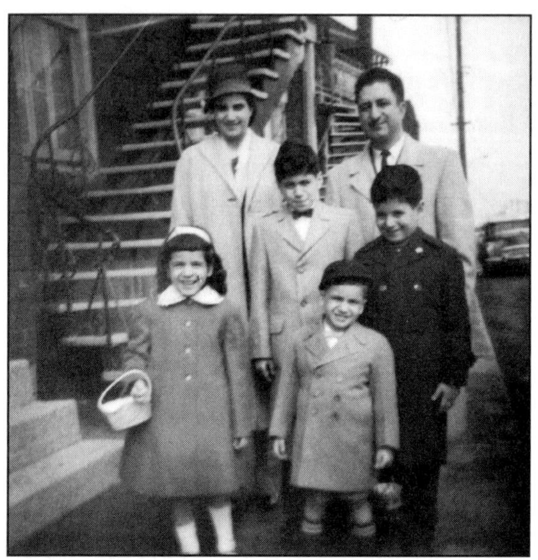

Growing up with parents John and Rhoda in Lachine, circa 1960

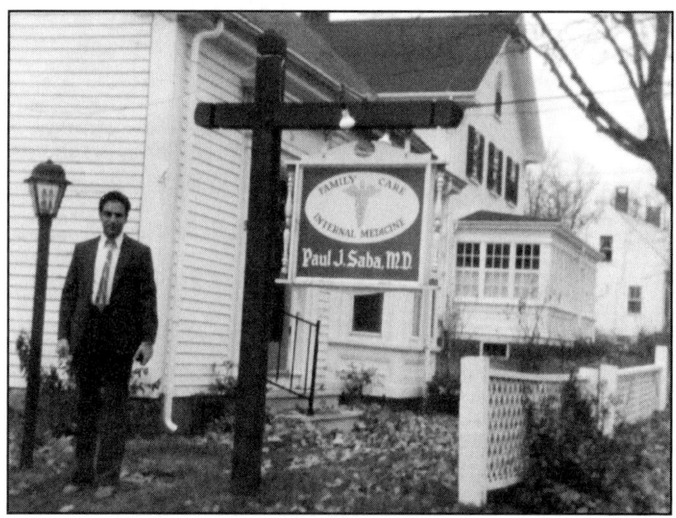

Working as a physician in Massachusetts

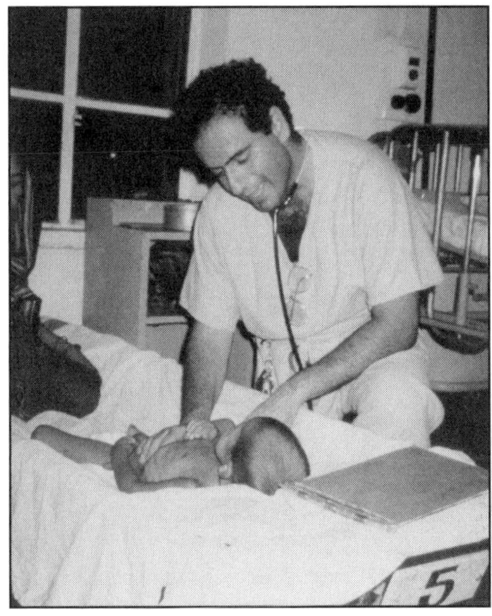

Caring for a child in Bangladesh, 1990

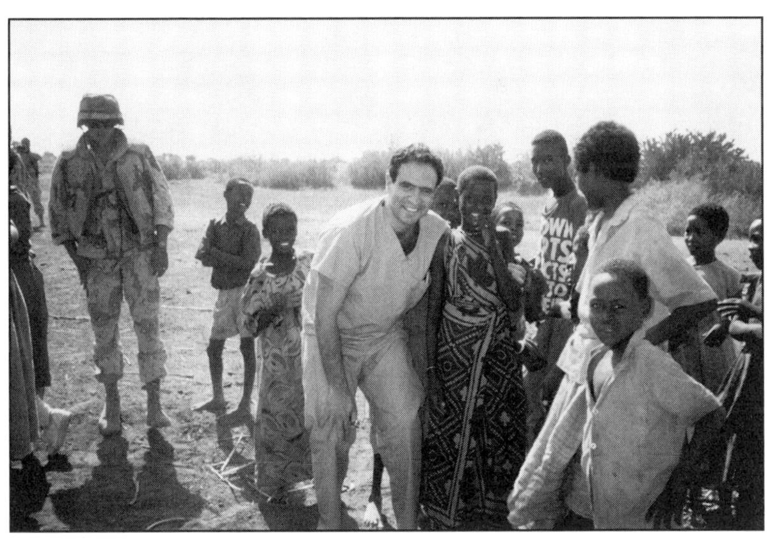

Part of the mobile health unit and UNOSOM forces in Somalia, 1993

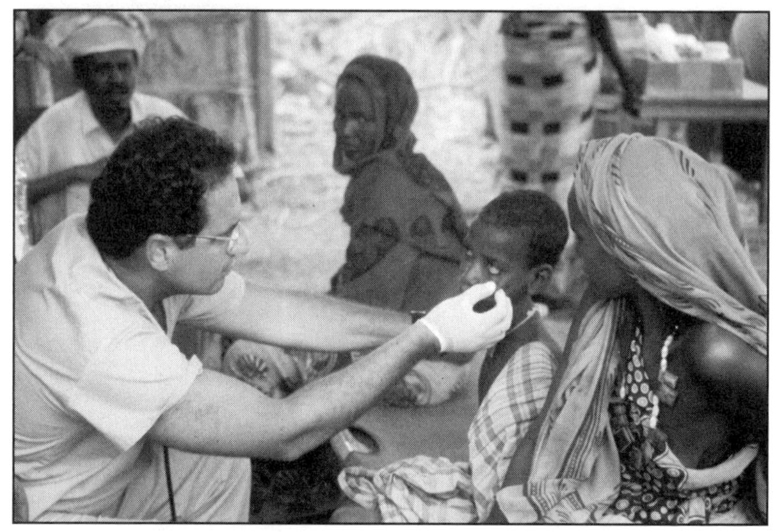

Caring for a child in Somalia, 1993

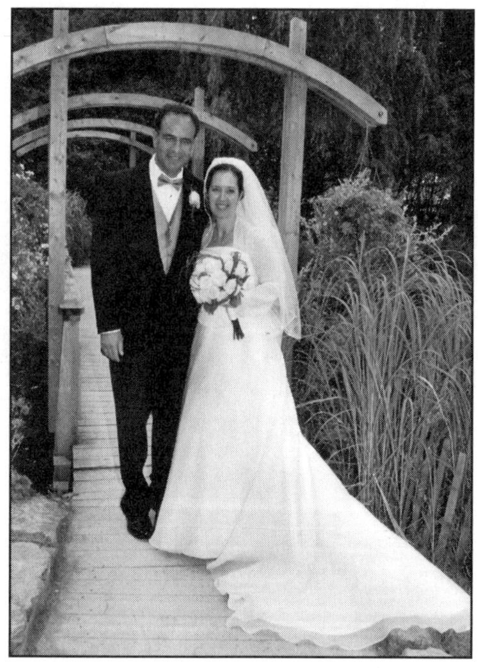

Newly wed at 50

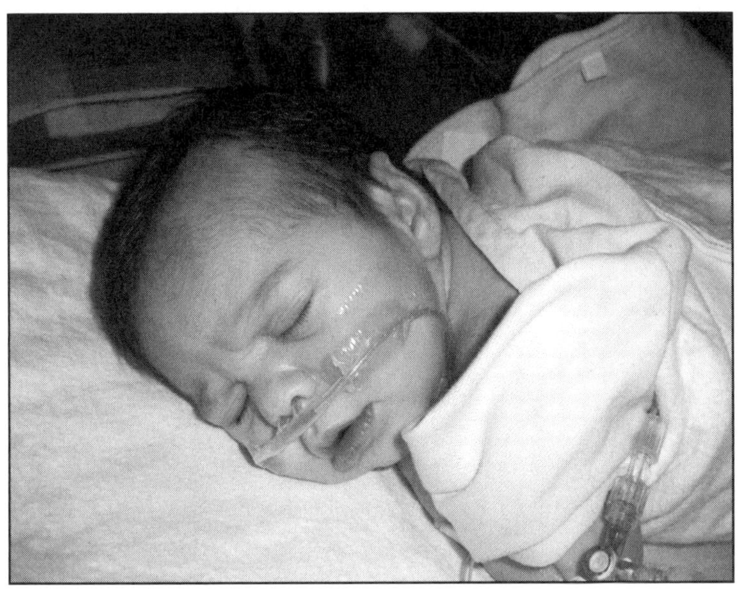

*Jessica in the neonatal intensive care unit
of Montreal Children's Hospital, 2009*

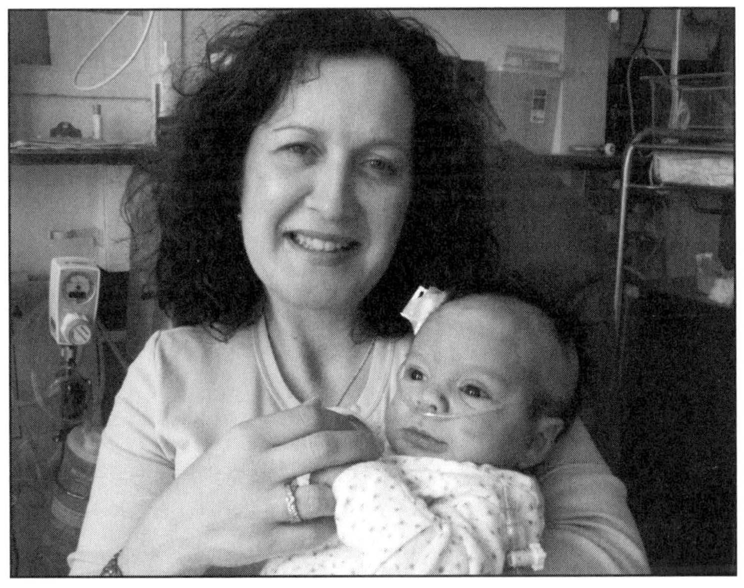

*Jessica and Mom in the neonatal intensive care unit
of Montreal Children's Hospital, 2009*

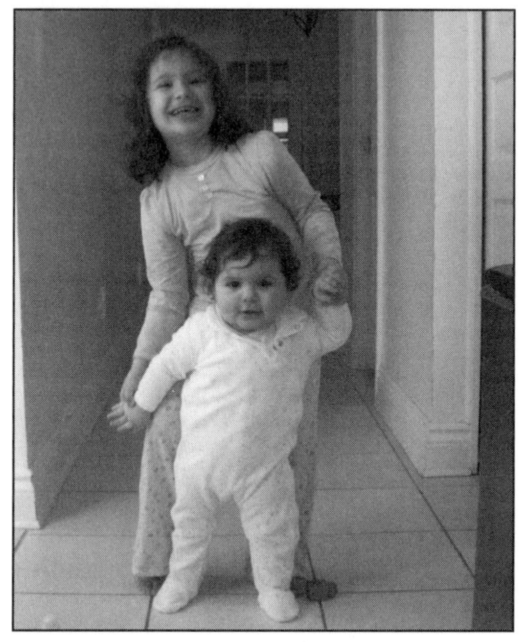

Jessica and Eliana at home dancing in their pajamas

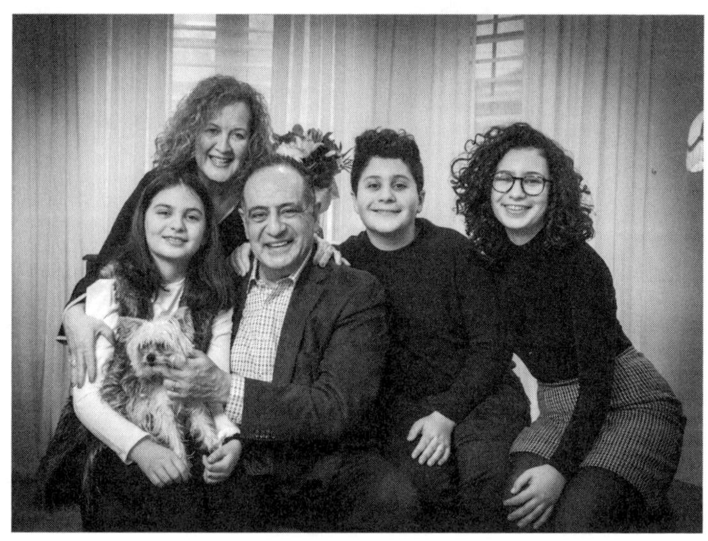

Saba family portrait, 2020

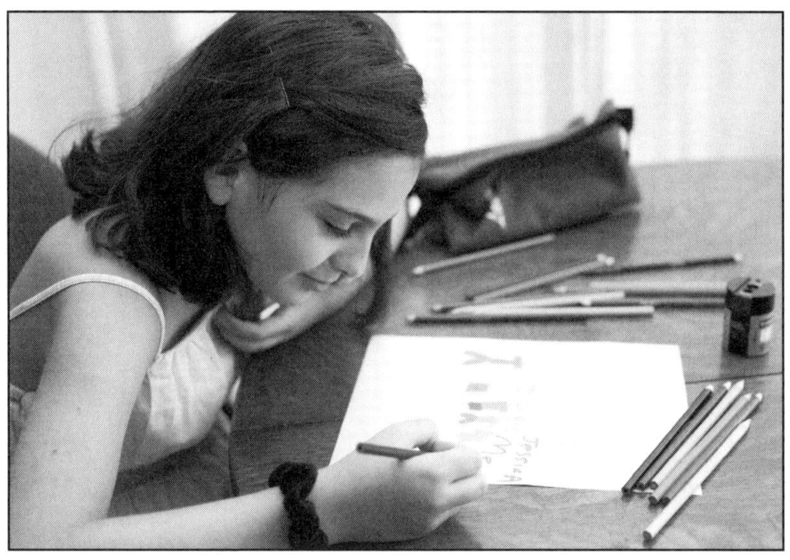

Jessica with her painting "Made to Live"

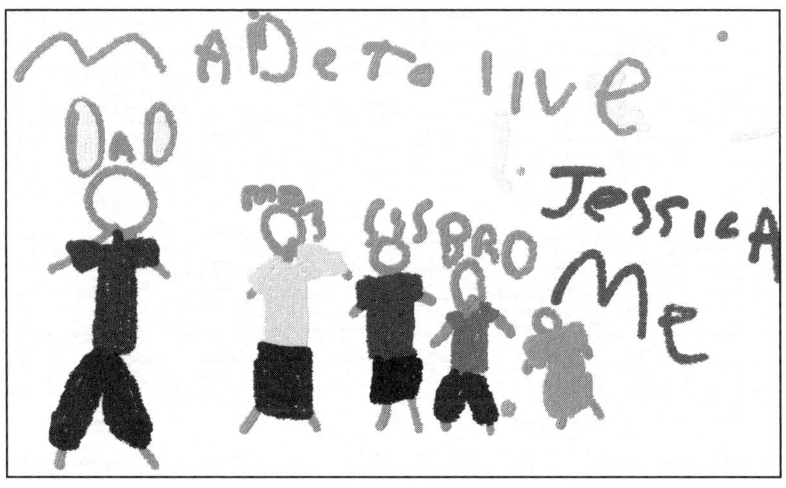

Jessica's painting "Made to Live"

CHAPTER 5

FIGHTING FOR LIFE

It can feel peculiar to appear before a judge in court fighting against your own democratically elected provincial government. Normally, if we imagine ourselves in front of a court, we think of it as resulting from an accusation that we've done something, either criminally or civilly. Alternatively, we might think of it as an outcome of events going terribly wrong in our lives: a divorce, for example, or a child custody dispute.

Whatever the cause, we hope and pray that we are never actually forced into court. I certainly never pictured myself taking legal action to try to stop my own government from enacting legislation that I knew in my heart as a doctor was dangerously wrong. Yet that is exactly where I found myself in the spring of 2014, seeking to prevent the Quebec government from proceeding with its euthanasia legislation.

From then until now, I've spent north of $150,000 engaging the legal system to fight the law. A small part of it has been offset by a few kind donors. For the rest, I had to sit down with my wife and decide whether to go ahead alone despite the effect on our family's finances. We decided it was worth it to fight.

Having gone through the process, it's reasonable to ask: was it worth it? My immediate answer is "yes," quickly followed by the proviso that I haven't yet given up the fight, despite my lawyer's counsel that the case really can't go much further except on a few specific issues. Whether it actually gets to the Supreme Court of Canada and we can reverse the decision or not—and in my wildest dreams I continue to hope it might happen—there are two specific outcomes that justify all the hope, time, energy, and yes, money.

The first outcome, which I alluded to in an earlier chapter, is that for a brief shining moment on December 1, 2015 we were able to stop the government's euthanasia juggernaut with a temporary injunction against proclaiming the law.[37] That might sound about as successful as hitting a grizzly bear with a flyswatter. Perhaps it was.

But after having been initially turned down in our attempt at an injunction, it felt an awful lot like victory, however short-lived it might have been. We even had the federal government on our side, because we were able to argue that there was a federal prohibition on killing by whatever means, and therefore the Quebec government could not pass a law that infringed on federal law.

Unfortunately for us, politics reared its grisly head. The Canadian government, led by the newly elected Prime Minister Justin Trudeau and the Attorney General, did an about-face, which was followed by our bright, shining victory being unceremoniously extinguished. At that time, according to Canada's major newspaper, "Ottawa has already indicated it sees value in Quebec's law. Prime Minister Justin Trudeau this month praised Quebec's 'responsible and rigorous approach to such a delicate and sensitive topic.'"[38]

---

[37] "Quebec End-of-Life Law Contradicts the Criminal Code and Can't Take Effect, Court Says," *CBC News*, December 1, 2015 (https://www.cbc.ca/news/canada/montreal/quebec-end-of-life-care-1.3345572).

[38] Ingrid Peretz, "Quebec's Right-to-Die Law Upheld by Court," *The Globe and Mail*, December 22, 2015 (https://www.theglobeandmail.com/news/national/quebec-government-wins-challenge-on-assisted-dying-law/article27901664/).

The Quebec government got its way, and its law was proclaimed at the end of December 2015. We had shown, though, that the courts could still be turned to for counterbalance against legislative error on euthanasia and assisted suicide. That, at least, was a source of hope.

We did not simply retreat defeated. We fought on in court, which brought about the second critical outcome of this legal battle. The Attorney General of Quebec (AGQ) even stated that I could not speak against euthanasia in the case because I am "not a supporter or defender of medical aid in dying." Morever, the AGQ declared that I should not be heard by the court because my intention is not to expand MAiD. Consequently, since I am opposed to MAiD I am not allowed to fight against euthanasia.[39] While that might seem overwhelmingly negative, it opened my eyes wide to how deeply the euthanasia and assisted suicide mentality had permeated the institutions of governance in Quebec and Canada, including the legislatures, the regulatory bodies, and even the courts, as a looming Supreme Court of Canada decision in the *Carter* case would ultimately show.

In February 2015, the Supreme Court overturned its own ruling from twenty-two years earlier and declared unconstitutional the section of the Canadian Criminal Code that made assisted suicide illegal. Within sixteen months of that ruling, the country was scrambling to implement the newly coined Medical Aid in Dying regime (MAiD).

Under the 2016 legislation,[40] euthanasia or assisted suicide is legal for those who "have a serious and incurable illness, disease or disability" and "are in an advanced state of irreversible decline

---

[39] Attorney General of Quebec, "Motion to Dismiss," April 20, 2017: Dr Saba c. PGQ-PGC/Dossier C.S. 500-17-082567-143, paragraphs 29–31.

[40] "Bill C-14," *Parliament of Canada.* June 17, 2016 (https://www.parl.ca/DocumentViewer/en/42-1/bill/C-14/royal-assent).

in capability," and "that illness, disease or disability or that state of decline causes them enduring physical or psychological suffering that is intolerable to them and that cannot be relieved under conditions that they consider acceptable."

Death must be deemed to be "reasonably foreseeable… [but] without a prognosis necessarily having been made as to the specific length of time that they have remaining."[41] Even if a patient's suffering can be alleviated by medical care, treatment of the suffering is not mandatory, and the person can go directly to euthanasia or assisted suicide if they prefer.

Many believe the federal law was deliberately drafted to allow the widest latitude possible for medically administered killing of patients. Just how wide?

That might be best exemplified by the example of Dr. Ellen Wiebe from British Columbia. She was exonerated in August 2019 for sneaking into a Jewish hospital and terminating the life of an elderly patient.

Using smuggled medical equipment, she killed the ninety-two-year-old resident in his room, despite the facility's administration expressly prohibiting medically delivered death on site because of potential trauma it could cause Holocaust survivors living there. The B.C. College of Physicians and Surgeons deemed she did nothing unethical or wrong under existing legal regulations.[42]

In my own province of Quebec, neither the government nor the Quebec College of Physicians have shown any intention of intervening against or sanctioning physicians who have performed euthanasia in non-conformity with the law. Moreover, the previous Liberal government commissioned experts "to look into

---

[41] Ibid.

[42] Alex Rose, "B.C. Doctor Cleared of Assisted Death in Jewish Home," *Canadian Jewish News*, Aug. 9, 2019 (https://www.cjnews.com/news/canada/b-c-doctor-cleared-of-assisted-death-in-jewish-home).

the 'complex question' of expanding the law to have it apply to people who are deemed 'legally and clinically unfit' to give consent to the procedure."[43]

The 2014 Quebec law and the 2016 federal law have similarities and differences. The commonality of both laws is that human life can be eliminated if the person makes a request, is considered to be suffering, and has a limited life term.

Under the provincial law, euthanasia must be available to adults who are at "the end of life" and suffer from "a serious and incurable illness; are in an advanced state of irreversible decline in capability; and experience constant and unbearable physical or psychological suffering which cannot be relieved in a manner the patient deems tolerable." The patient requesting medical aid in dying must do so "in a free and informed manner."[44] As we saw in the previous chapter, pressures ranging from hospital cost-cutting to patient fear of suffering can interfere with any MAiD request coming close to qualifying as free, informed, and consensual.

As a Quebec doctor, I am not forced to administer the lethal injection that kills someone subjected to MAiD. I am, however, forced to refer my patient to "the executive director of the institution" to "ensure continuity of care."[45] Continuity of *care* will deliberately end with the patient being dead, of course. Neither the Quebec government nor the province's chief medical regulatory body nor the legal system seem concerned with such an oxymoronic transformation of the meaning of healthcare.

On the contrary, the Quebec Human Rights Commission and Youth Protection Commission has recommended extending

---

[43] Giuseppe Valiante, "More than 600 Cases of Doctor-Assisted Death in Quebec in 2016–17," *National Post*, October 26, 2017.

[44] "Loi Concernant les soins de Fin de Vie," *Légis Québec*, Sept. 1, 2019 (http://legisquebec.gouv.qc.ca/fr/ShowDoc/cs/S-32.0001).

[45] Ibid.

euthanasia to children.[46] Next door in Ontario, the Advisory Group on Physician-Assisted Dying Health Board also recommended extending euthanasia to children. Children could see their lives ended prematurely without parental consent or prior notification.[47]

In December 2016, the Canadian Council of Academies (CCA) was asked by the Canadian government to undertake independent reviews related to three types of MAiD requests: by mature minors, advance requests, and requests where a mental disorder is the sole underlying medical condition.

In December 2018, the CCA released the three final reports, one on each type of request. While there were no explicit recommendations, in a chapter on children near the end of the report, there is wording that suggests bias towards childhood euthanasia:

> Despite research demonstrating that some minors are capable of making critical healthcare decisions, including end-of-life choices, some argue that minors as a group are too vulnerable to be given the ability to request MAID.
>
> However, part of protecting potentially vulnerable patients is to ensure that they are listened to. Thus, it has been argued that, rather than denying healthcare choices to groups frequently labelled as vulnerable, society must provide the accommodations to ensure that everyone is protected not only from exploitation, but also from being ignored and excluded.[48]

---

[46] "Mémoire à la Commission de la Santé et des Services Sociaux De L'Assemblée Nationale: Projet De Loi N° 52, Loi Concernant Les Soins De Fin De Vie," *Commission des Droites de la Personne et des Droits de la Jeunesse Québec*, September 2013 (http://www.cdpdj.qc.ca/Publications/memoire_PL52_soins-fin-de-vie.pdf).

[47] "Final Report," *Provincial-Territorial Expert Advisory Group on Physician-Assisted Dying*, November 30, 2015 (http://www.health.gov.on.ca/en/news/bulletin/2015/docs/eagreport_20151214_en.pdf).

[48] Council of Canadian Academies, *The State of Knowledge on Medical Assistance in Dying for Mature Minors* (Ottawa, ON: The Expert Panel Working Group on MAID for Mature Minors, Council of Canadian Academies, 2018).

So, in the foreseeable future in Canada, it's possible that children will be protected from feeling ignored or excluded in order for their bodies to be injected with a lethal drug that will stop their beating hearts and kill them. Do you begin to see why my eyes have opened so wide since the beginning of my legal fight against MAiD?

Perhaps most frightening of all is that the path lying before Canada and Quebec is already so evident in the Netherlands and in Belgium, where the terrible doctrines and practices of euthanasia and assisted suicide emerged first in the post-war world. In both countries, child euthanasia is tolerated or has been legalized. In the Netherlands, one in two hundred infants dies within the first year of life. Sixty percent of these deaths are preceded by an end-of-life decision.[49]

In Belgium, a nine-year-old and an eleven-year-old have reportedly been euthanized. The eleven-year-old had cystic fibrosis, "a congenital respiratory disease that is incurable and fatal, but which modern treatments have enabled many patients to enjoy high quality of life well into their 30s or even beyond…"[50] According to Cystic Fibrosis Canada, the median age of survival is fifty-two years.[51]

As CTV News has reported, just recently a new treatment for cystic fibrosis called Trikafta has been approved in the United States. Considered "miraculous," the treatment "fixes that defective protein rather than just treating the symptoms." According to the report,

> For CF patients like 28-year-old Esiason, the new drug means thinking about life long-term. …

---

[49] P. Voultsos & F. Chatzinikolaou, "Involuntary Euthanasia of Severely Ill Newborns: Is the Groningen Protocol Really Dangerous?," *Hippokratia* 18, no. 3 (2014): 193–203.

[50] Charles Lane, "Children Are Being Euthanized in Belgium," *Washington Post*, Aug. 6, 2018.

[51] See https://www.cysticfibrosis.ca/our-programs/cf-registry.

"When you're living with a terminal illness, you kind of live day to day," said Esiason. "As soon as my health turned around, it was like, 'OK, what am I going to do next? I'm really looking forward to the rest of my life because of this amazing breakthrough."[52]

The pharmaceutical company Vertex "has also submitted the triple therapy [Trikafta] to the European Medicines Agency, with a decision expected in 2020."[53] What if the children who were euthanized in Belgium had been able to hang on a little longer until this new drug was developed? Unfortunately, in Canada this life-saving drug is not yet available and it may be years before it is approved, which will cost needless suffering and loss of life.[54]

These are bleak realities indeed. Yet, as with our small moment of triumph in getting the law delayed, there are countervailing points of light that can help cultivate optimism and even hope. One of them comes from California, of all places, where the state's assisted suicide law was temporarily overturned by a superior court judge in 2018.[55]

Although the End of Life Option Act was later upheld, the initial victory gave Dr. David Stevens, executive director of the American Academy of Medical Ethics, a chance to tell CNN's audience that the legislation "isn't about giving patients the right

[52] Jonathan Forani, "'Miracle' Cystic Fibrosis Drug Approved in U.S., Canadian Trials Underway," *CTV News*, Oct. 29, 2019 (https://beta.ctvnews.ca/national/health/2019/10/29/1_4660328.html).

[53] Lucy Parsons, "Vertex Scores FDA Approval for CF Triple Therapy Trikafta," *PMLive.com*, Oct. 22, 2019 (https://www.pmlive.com/pharma_news/vertex_scores_fda_approval_of_cf_triple_therapy_trikafta_1314110).

[54] Matt Gilmour & Adam Kovac, "'This Drug Saved My Life': Cystic Fibrosis Patient Accuses Drug Company, Canada of Stalling on Approval," *CTV News*, November 17, 2019 (https://montreal.ctvnews.ca/this-drug-saved-my-life-cystic-fibrosis-patient-accuses-drug-company-canada-of-stalling-on-approval-1.4689924).

[55] Susan Scutti, "California Judge Overturns Ed of Life Option Law, *CNN.com*, May 16, 2018 (https://www.cnn.com/2018/05/16/health/california-assisted-suicide-law-overturned/index.html).

to die. This is about giving doctors the right to assist in killing…. [It] is dangerous for the healthcare profession. It destroys trust between the doctor and the patient…. [And] the so-called right to die very quickly becomes the duty to die."[56]

In another media report, Alexandra Snyder, executive director of the Life Legal Defense Foundation, said the ruling "reinstates critical legal protections for vulnerable patients…. The court made it very clear that assisted suicide has nothing to do with increasing access to healthcare and that hijacking the special session to advance an unrelated agenda is impermissible."[57]

Stephanie Packer, whose insurance company refused her life-saving chemotherapy treatment and offered $1.20 worth of "aid-in-dying" drugs instead, made the point through various media channels that "Choice is really an illusion for a very few. For too many, assisted suicide will be the only affordable 'treatment' that is offered them."[58]

These might seem small steps indeed on the very long road back from euthanasia and assisted suicide regimes that now extend to children as young as nine years old—or younger. But we did not get so far down in a single bound, either.

From its origins in the eugenics movement of the early twentieth century through the nightmare of the Holocaust and the incessant breaking down of Judeo-Christian ethics and understanding over the past two generations, the euthanasia and assisted suicide movement settled in early for the long haul. It has worn and wormed its way into our most important institutions, into the foundations of legal and medical thinking, into the very

---

[56] Ibid.

[57] Dennis Romero & Associated Press, "Judge Overturns California's Doctor-Assisted Suicide Law," *NBC News*, May 15, 2018 (https://www.nbcnews.com/news/crime-courts/judge-overturns-california-s-doctor-assisted-suicide-law-n874486).

[58] Catholic News Agency, "Judge Rules California Assisted Suicide Law Was Wrongfully Rushed," May 16, 2018 (https://www.catholicnewsagency.com/news/judge-rules-california-assisted-suicide-law-was-wrongfully-rushed-97100).

way we have been misled to think about suffering, and about life itself.

Yet my legal fight against the Quebec euthanasia law is but one of many initiatives, led by stalwart campaigners, that will provide first the resistance, then the lawful revision, and ultimately the elimination of legislation enshrining euthanasia and assisted suicide. During the summer of 2019, for example, Alex Schadenberg marked twenty years as the executive director of the Euthanasia Prevention Coalition, which has consistently fought alongside groups such as Physicans for Life, the Christian Medical Dental Association, and the Christian Legal Foundation against the culture of death in Canada.

"I started doing this because I looked around and didn't see anyone else doing it," Alex Schadenberg told Convivium magazine[59] in August 2019. "I have to keep involved…. The reality is, you can't be silent. You can't be silent about a law that allows physicians and nurse practitioners to kill people. I have no fear of death. I do fear a country that allows people to kill me."

We are all called, in our various capacities and to the best of our abilities, to turn fear into hope. That means turning Canada, once again, into a country where we remember that we are made to live.

---

[59] Peter Stockland, "MAiD in Canada," *Convivium*, August 9, 2019 (https://www. convivium.ca/articles/maid-in-canada).

Chapter 6
A Long History of Devaluing Life

So far, this book has used the terms euthanasia, assisted suicide and Medical Aid in Dying without specifically defining them. One reason is that the phrases have become so intermingled and interchangeable that it's almost more confusing to try to set them back to their original meanings. Another reason is that debates over the technical meaning of the terms can be used as a kind of smokescreen around what is really being done: the intentional premature killing of a human being before the natural physical processes of the body release their hold on life. Like many who have battled the medical termination mindset, I strongly believe this confusion of terminology has been a deliberate distraction ploy to obscure the reality of what is being done. This confusion of language is described by the Canadian psychologist Albert Bandura as sanitizing "euphemistic language." According to Fabrian Stahle, "It is all about verbal engineering [euthanasia proponents use] to convince themselves, as well as to influence general opinion, that something which initially fills most people with a sense of disgust is in fact something indicative of high moral standards."[60]

---

[60] Fabian Stahle, "Moral Disengagement—Mechanisms Propelling the Euthanasia/PAS Movement," *Journal of Ethics in Mental Health* 10 (2017): 1.

Manipulation of language has historically led to great moral depravities. Proponents of euthanasia, assisted suicide, and MAiD have scored a significant propaganda victory by creating the impression that what they advocate is progress, that they are advancing history in new and never-before-imagined gestures of human openness, tolerance, and respect. As Stahle writes,

> There is a gradual slide downwards in moral depravity and justification of killing another human being. It begins with a moral justification; the patient should not have to suffer. It continues with some euphemisms; it is a dignified death, it is aid-in-dying and absolutely not suicide. Finally, there is the exonerative comparison; it is much better than that the patient should take his/her own life.[61]

In fact, the current regimes legalizing intentional medical killing of patients are the living proof of Sir Winston Churchill's 1948 warning to the British House of Commons: "Those who fail to learn from history are doomed to repeat it."

Historically, **euthanasia**—often translated as "a good death"—occurs when one person requests, or is deemed to have consented to, having his or her life ended by a second person. Most commonly today, euthanasia is performed by a doctor or other healthcare professional injecting a lethal substance into the vein of the person being euthanized. Historically, however, numerous means have been used to euthanize. And as we saw in the previous chapter, it's far from unknown to provide euthanasia for children, or even the mentally ill, who lack all capacity to request and consent.

Assisted suicide is distinguished from euthanasia in that the person dies at his or her own hand, though after being given the

---

[61] Ibid, p. 1.

necessary means to cause death. A doctor, for example, would prescribe a type of medication that the individual would then pick up from the pharmacy, take home, and ingest. One of the novelties of the *Carter* decision referred to in an earlier chapter was the Supreme Court of Canada's acceptance of arguments that the federal law being challenged represented a form of discrimination because it "forced" people to commit suicide prematurely.

In short, Canada's highest court found existing prohibitions on assisted suicide meant that someone suffering from, say, Lou Gehrig's Disease would have to commit suicide on their own in an early stage of their illness before they became too incapacitated. This was deemed to violate Charter Rights protecting individual liberty. It seems never to have occurred to the Court that the better outcome would be for healthcare providers to ensure there's no need for suicide at all. As Fabian Stahl observes:

> The court was unable, or rather unwilling, to realize the ironic consequence of its decision – that such legalization has the exact opposite effect, as it will most likely cause a far greater number of individuals to take their lives prematurely with the help of doctors, than the number that would have done so completely independently in the same situation. When you use this exonerative comparison, it is also a denial of the fact that a wish to die most often is an expression of depression that can be treated with far better methods than a lethal prescription.[62]

Far from being a bold step forward on the road to progress, the *Carter* decision returned Canada to the state of Roman times,

---

[62] Ibid.

when the earliest written legislation, known as the Twelve Tables,[63] ordered the killing of deformed children. According to Table Four, "A dreadfully deformed child shall be quickly killed."[64] Like the nine justices of the Canadian Supreme Court who opened the door to Medical Aid in Dying, the Romans saw the abolition of the whole person as a legitimate answer to general human imperfections or specific forms of suffering.

The Roman philosophers known as Stoics, exemplified by Seneca, encouraged suicide for the elderly, poor, disabled, those with failing physical or mental health, the weary, and those for whom life was no longer deemed worthy. Self-destruction was considered to be an obligation to friends, family, and society. Killing oneself exhibited freedom and autonomy and preserved dignity, according to Seneca.

The Roman worldview was radically changed by Judeo-Christian philosophy that placed value on the intrinsic value of each human life and the prohibition to kill. The story of the Good Samaritan who stopped and aided a total stranger left for dead, as recounted by Jesus in the Gospel of Luke (10:25–37), exemplified the model of caring. It is often considered to be the foundation for modern day human rights legislation and the model for social and health measures enacted to protect children, the disabled, disadvantaged, and elderly, as well as those facing physical or mental challenges.

In Roman times, Christians cared for the sick, disabled, and dying. When the plague hit Carthage in the second century, Christians cared for those who were thrown out of their homes and left to die in the street. During the fourth century, Christians built hospices, which were guest houses for the sick and the disabled.

---

[63] "Law of the Twelve Tables," *Encyclopedia Brittanica* (https://www.britannica.com/topic/Law-of-the-Twelve-Tables).

[64] "The Law of the Twelve Tables" (http://thelatinlibrary.com/law/12tables.html).

Up to about 1000 A.D., hospitals were attached to cathedrals. This movement continued in the Middle Ages with the opening of monastic infirmaries and public hospitals.

During the eighteenth century, the "Age of Hospitals" was supported by Christian philanthropists; this movement spread from Europe to the New World. It continued during the Industrial Revolution of the nineteenth century. The Salvation Army, founded by William Booth, is an example of the outreach of medical care for the poor in urban areas.

The Sisters of Providence were known for their works of charity for the poor, indigenous, immigrants, disabled, those with mental health problems, women, and children, and their convictions led them to establish clinics and hospitals around the world that still exist today. St. Joseph's Hospital, where I work in Lachine, was founded by the Sisters[65] in 1913.

During the twentieth century, the modern-day hospice care movement was founded. An article on the website of the Christian Medical Fellowship[66] notes that, "Dame Cicely Saunders founded St Christopher's Hospice in 1967, with the aim of providing as peaceful an atmosphere as possible for those in their terminal illness, while offering an environment of Christian love and support."

Much of modern clinical medicine was advanced by Christian physicians, including the ethics of medical practice. Sir William Osler, who is considered by many as the father of modern medicine, emphasized bedside teaching and listening to patients to make the correct diagnosis. He graduated from McGill University's Faculty of Medicine in Montreal, and established himself for a time at the Montreal General Hospital. He later helped found Johns Hopkins Medical School.

[65] See https://providenceintl.org/en/ for information on the order.

[66] Rosie Beal-Preston, "The Christian Contribution to Medicine," *Christian Medical Fellowship* (2000) (https://www.cmf.org.uk/resources/publications/content/?context=article&id=827).

Osler was deeply influenced by Sir Thomas Browne, a seventeenth-century Christian physician who expanded on the Hippocratic principles and was one of the first to write on medical ethics and whole-person care. Sir William Osler "taught all medical students to base their attitudes and care for their patients on the standards laid down in the Bible."[67]

All of these movements away from the Roman attitudes toward life and death find their home in Jesus' teaching in the parable of the Good Samaritan about our obligations to others. Even those who, for whatever reason, disavow such a directly Christian directive must still contend with their entirely secular counterpart. In his oath[68] for physicians, the father of Western medicine, Hippocrates, forbade the giving of deadly medicine to any one if asked for it—nor were doctors even permitted to counsel euthanasia or what we now call assisted suicide.

Still, throughout my involvement in the battle against medical killing, I keep hearing the insistent claim: That was then; this is now. History is nice, the argument goes. But we've moved on from those stories of the past. We are post-Christian. We are no longer bound by the taboos of earlier, darker, superstitious ages.

We need only to consider the use of those very same claims in Germany through the 1930s up to 1945 to see how dangerously, seductively wrong they are. Of course, referring to that horrifying era of history carries dangers itself because it risks being accused of comparing contemporary proponents of euthanasia, assisted suicide, and MAiD to the Nazis. Of course, to suggest such a thing would be a horrible calumny against them. They are not like the Nazis. The Nazis were like them, just as the Nazis were like all of us.

---

[67] Ibid.

[68] "Hippocratic Oath," *Encyclopedia Brittanica* (https://www.britannica.com/topic/Hippocratic-oath).

Guilty as they were of historically monstrous atrocities, the Nazis were not sons and daughters of Dr. Frankenstein. They were not laboratory-created monsters. They were human beings drawn, through terribly deluded thinking, into committing all the vile, evil acts that Judeo-Christianity—and indeed many faith traditions—have spoken against for millennia. As the philosopher Hannah Arendt wrote in the 1960s, they were not, as individuals, fundamentally evil.[69] They were flesh-and-blood banalities trapped by varying mixtures of greed, ambition, cowardice, moral shortsightedness, and lust for power into a vortex from which escape became almost impossible, and death the solution to every problem.

That inability to return to the light from the darkness of a death-dealing ideology is what connects the current proponents of medical killing to their historical antecedents. The common link is not one of evil. It is going down a path that by its nature quickly reaches a point of no return.

Dealing medical death does not just make medical death desirable or even necessary. It makes it unavoidable. To acknowledge the first medical death as wrong would have been to admit an ideological error. To acknowledge it as wrong after more than thirteen thousand deaths—the toll for MAiD in Canada since 2016[70]—would be to admit to mass murder. In a great paradox, the higher the death count, the more impossible it becomes to admit the death count is significant. Or in the words infamously attributed to Josef Stalin, "One man dying of hunger is a tragedy. A million dying of hunger is a statistic."

Yet the increasing difficulty of pushing back against the moral inertia of legalized euthanasia, assisted suicide, and MAiD does

---

[69] Hannah Arendt, *Eichmann in Jerusalem: A Report on the Banality of Evil* (New York: Viking, 1963).

[70] This is according to statistics released on February 24, 2020 by the federal government. https://www.canada.ca/en/department-justice/news/2020/02/government-of-canada-proposes-changes-to-medical-assistance-in-dying-legislation.html

not exempt those of us opposed from speaking out and battling it by every peaceful means available. The German pastor Dietrich Bonhoeffer gave us the reason: "Not to speak is to speak. Not to act is to act."[71] Bonhoeffer, of course, was executed on April 9, 1945 for his part in a plot to assassinate Hitler after spending the war years valiantly speaking out and acting against the outrages of the Nazi regime.

Few (if any) of us will face such a history-defining fate. But there are ways we can all confront the medical killing juggernaut during the ordinary course of our lives. One of them is simply what you are doing right now: reading books like this one to become, or keep yourself, informed on the issue itself—its status, legal challenges to it, the most current arguments against it, groups you might be able in some way to help continue the battle. A second is to engage your neighbours attentively, respectfully, and charitably to gently correct one or two misconceptions they might have about what euthanasia, assisted suicide, and MAiD really mean.

Although I do a lot of media work, give speeches, and write publicly against medical killing, my most precious venue is the chance to communicate to my patients my opposition to euthanasia, assisted suicide, and MAiD. Of course, I always communicate in a way that accords those patients their full recognition as independent adults who have the capacity to make their own decisions. They must be able to trust me to do that, and they do.

Indeed, my patients come to me because they trust me. They trust that I will act in their best interests and not my own. That I will provide the best in medical care. That I will neither mislead them nor short-change them. That I will care.

---

[71] Emily Maust Wood, "20 Influential Quotes by Dietrich Bonhoeffer," *Crosswalk*, Nov. 23, 2015 (https://www.crosswalk.com/faith/spiritual-life/inspiring-quotes/20-influential-quotes-by-dietrich-bonhoeffer.html).

I will cure sometimes, alleviate suffering always. But I will not kill. They know that up front. It is a basic contract between us based on trust and respect.

Euthanasia and assisted suicide *do* kill. They are state-sanctioned killing. They are wrong, and they remain wrong whether the state sanctions them or not. They are not medicine. They cause needless loss of life. It is wrong to kill people even when they request it.

As mentioned earlier, in Quebec I am not required by law to euthanize, but I am required to refer patients to be euthanized. In the province of Ontario, physicians through a court judgement are being forced to participate by referral, but are in the process of appealing that judgement. However, in the province of Manitoba, physicians are not forced to participate.[72]

It is noteworthy that in the United States of America, according to the *Wall Street Journal*, "The Trump administration will expand enforcement of protections for medical workers with moral or faith-based objections to medical procedures such as abortion [and] assisted suicide…. The rule is needed, supporters say, because many health-care providers have long felt they have had to violate their beliefs and often lack the ability to bring legal action on their own."[73] Unfortunately, this executive order was overturned by a New York federal judge. Physicians' rights of conscientious objection risk being infringed upon, unless there is an appeal by the Trump administration.[74]

---

[72] Government of Manitoba, "Bill 34: The Medical Assistance in Dying (Protection for Health Professionals and Others) Act" (https://web2.gov.mb.ca/bills/41-2/pdf/b034.pdf).

[73] Stephanie Armour, "White House Unveils Rule to Protect Health Workers' Religious, Moral Beliefs," *Wall Street Journal*, May 28, 2019 (https://www.wsj.com/articles/white-house-unveils-rules-to-protect-health-workers-religious-moral-beliefs-11556816255).

[74] Stephanie Armour, "Federal Judge Strikes Down Rule on Conscience Provisions for Medical Providers," *Wall Street Journal*, November 6, 2019 (https://www.wsj.com/articles/federal-judge-strikes-down-rule-on-conscience-provisions-for-medical-providers-11573064086).

In Quebec, I am forced to participate, but I refuse to participate. I refuse because I did not become a doctor to kill. As a doctor, husband, father, and Christian, I do not believe we were made to kill or be killed. We were, I firmly believe, made to live.

CHAPTER 7

FIGHTING FOR LIFE INTERNATIONALLY

In the previous chapter, I cited philosopher Hannah Arendt's insight that the vast majority of the Nazi hierarchy who committed unspeakable crimes against humanity were not laboratory-created monsters, but banal humans made mad by ambition, vanity, and lust for power. Arendt's commentary in works such as *Eichmann in Jerusalem* and *The Origins of Totalitarianism* echoes the declaration of psychiatrist Viktor E. Frankl, himself a Holocaust survivor, on the root causes of such evil deformation of personhood.

"I am absolutely convinced," Frankl wrote, "that the gas chambers of Auschwitz, Treblinka, and Maidanek were ultimately prepared not in some ministry or other in Berlin, but rather at the desks and lecture halls of nihilistic scientists and philosophers."[75]

To trace a source of inhumanity, however, is not to excuse or exonerate the people who undertake heinous acts. The principle was vigorously affirmed during the Nuremberg trials that followed the Second World War, where former Nazi leaders were indicted and tried as war criminals. Individuals could not use the "superior orders" defence or argue that they were compelled by an "act of

---

[75] Available at https://www.goodreads.com/quotes/7322711-if-we-present-a-man-with-a-concept-of-man.

state" in following orders that a country or a state had enacted. *Perspectives on the Nuremberg Trial,*[76] edited by Guénaël Mettraux, lays out the seven principles that emerged from the proceedings. Principle number four is explicit in placing responsibility on the individual who carries out an act that can be deemed criminal or a crime against humanity.

"The fact that a person acted pursuant to order of his Government or of a superior does not relieve him from responsibility under international law, provided a moral choice was in fact possible to him," it reads.[77]

The Nuremberg principles formed part of the basis of international law when "The General Assembly (of the United Nations) directed the International Law Commission to formulate the principles of international law recognized at the Nuremberg trials, in which German war criminals were prosecuted, and to prepare a draft code of offenses against the peace and security of mankind. In 1950 the commission submitted its formulation of the Nuremberg principles, which covered crimes against peace, war crimes, and crimes against humanity."[78]

Intriguingly, during Nuremberg, it was demonstrated that endorsing, referring, or acquiescing to euthanasia made one an accomplice to euthanasia, and this was considered a crime. The result of the Nuremberg principles, their enshrinement in the formulation of international law, and the explicit inclusion of reference to euthanasia finds expression today in the World Medical Association stipulation that the procedure is contrary to medical ethics.

---

[76] Guénaël Mettraux, *Perspectives on the Nuremberg Trial* (Oxford: Oxford University Press, 2008).

[77] "Principles of International Law Recognized in the Charter of the Nürnberg Tribunal and in the Judgment of the Tribunal," *Yearbook of the International Law Commission* 2 (1950): para. 97 (https://kozidryngiel.files.wordpress.com/2009/01/nuremberg-principles.pdf).

[78] "United Nations: Development of International Law," *Encyclopedia Brittanica* (https://www.britannica.com/topic/United-Nations/The-environment).

The WMA, which represents more than ten million doctors in 112 countries, strongly encourages doctors to refuse to participate in an act of euthanasia and physician-assisted sucide, even where permitted by national law. In October 2019, the WMA updated its Declaration on Euthanasia and Physician-Assisted Suicide, which now reads as follows:

> The WMA reiterates its strong commitment to the principles of medical ethics and that utmost respect has to be maintained for human life. Therefore, the WMA is firmly opposed to euthanasia and physician-assisted suicide.
>
> For the purpose of this declaration, euthanasia is defined as a physician deliberately administering a lethal substance or carrying out an intervention to cause the death of a patient with decision-making capacity at the patient's own voluntary request. Physician-assisted suicide refers to cases in which, at the voluntary request of a patient with decision-making capacity, a physician deliberately enables a patient to end his or her own life by prescribing or providing medical substances with the intent to bring about death.
>
> No physician should be forced to participate in euthanasia or assisted suicide, nor should any physician be obliged to make referral decisions to this end.
>
> Separately, the physician who respects the basic right of the patient to decline medical treatment does not act unethically in forgoing or withholding unwanted care, even if respecting such a wish results in death of the patient.[79]

---

[79] World Medical Association, "WMA Declaration on Euthanasia and Physician-Assisted Suicide," Oct. 27, 2019 (https://www.wma.net/policies-post/declaration-on-euthanasia-and-physician-assisted-suicide/).

Of course, as a democratic, widely-dispersed, and entirely voluntary association, no one in the World Medical Association has visions of Nuremberg-style hearings to determine physician complicity in countries where euthanasia and medical killing have been legalized. What's important, though, is that the WMA takes the Nuremberg principle of individual agency and responsibility as a serious element of medical ethics. It reminds the more than ten million doctors who are its members that they have both the prerogative and the responsibility to say "no" to euthanasia, assisted suicide, and MAiD. It keeps them aware that these procedures are not ethical medicine, no matter what national governments might say on a purely legal level.

That is part of the reason that working with and through the WMA at international meetings has been an important complement to my domestic battle against medical killing in Canada. The other part is that, almost from the beginning of my medical career, I saw overseas doctoring as an important part of my own practice—and a working out of my Christian faith.

In my last year of residency in internal medicine, the civil war in Lebanon was going on, and I was quite touched by the stories about the children who had burns. I met up with an insurance agent named Robert who was a member of the Shriners and was helping get burn victims into the Shriners Hospital. Through a group affiliated with Oxfam America, I organized doctors and nurses to go there.

I created an organization called Medical Network for Lebanon Relief, and was able to take a month off and go to a village in the southern part of Lebanon to organize medical relief. It was a Shia Muslim village, so of course when I went there, the villagers were very suspicious of me. They couldn't understand why a non-Muslim person would come and help them. First, they thought I was an Israeli spy. Then they thought maybe I was a Palestinian infiltrator. I told them that I just really, really wanted to help.

It worked, and the clinic we set up worked for many years. We saw people with all types of medical problems. Sometimes they would try to come in with guns, saying they wanted to ensure that the patient was taken care of. I absolutely refused to allow the guns inside the clinic. I guess I was pretty brave in those days.

Each day around 4 p.m. we had to close the clinic for prayer. The only way to have their prayer broadcast was with the help of a gas generator, and for some reason it had to be put inside the room where the clinic was held. I never learned why it couldn't be put outside, but we'd have to close and that would be the end of the clinic day.

This was in 1983, just before the U.S. Embassy was bombed. Traveling from Beirut to the south of Lebanon and going through towns that had been hit by the civil war helped me see early on how medical help, medical relief, crossed all political boundaries. There were no political lines. We went to help people.[80]

It was my first experience of learning that we have to help people, and at the time it was based on humanistic values, because I considered myself agnostic. Here were these amazing people—from people doing relief work to Marines doing peacekeeping—working in very difficult, dangerous situations and willing to put their lives at stake to help.

We are all responsible for our actions as human beings. At the same time, some part of us makes us want to extend ourselves to other people, to make it our responsibility to ensure they are safe, housed, fed, given medical treatment, and able to pray in their own fashion. It often seems to me we are made as much to give as we are made to live.

---

[80] I recounted the story in the *Duxbury Clipper* in an article published on December 22, 1983 entitled "The Clipper Visits Dr. Paul Saba."

In a very simple but precise way, that pinpoints the wrong of treating euthanasia or assisted suicide as medicine. In such procedures, doctors give an injection whose entire purpose is the taking of life. But real medicine is about giving back to the patient as much as possible of what the patient once had—health, mobility, security—even life itself in the case of emergency procedures. It is not about giving something that explicitly takes away the most important thing the patient has always had: Life itself.

This is borne out by my international experiences in medicine, beginning in Lebanon. Like most of those around me, I was there to give medical attention to those in need. I wasn't thinking of my own life being in danger. One day, I was wandering around on a little tour of the village and my nurse began calling to me, "Get out. Don't move." He came and got me and guided me back to safety. Only then did I learn there were anti-personnel bombs placed throughout the village. Who knew? I sure didn't. I learned in that moment, though, that giving still requires practicing the virtue of prudence.

In a neighbouring town called Marjayoun, I met an Israeli lieutenant colonel who helped us transfer a Muslim patient having a seizure that I couldn't get under control. The Israelis let us cross the border into Israel so we could get to a hospital. Again, the humanitarian values crossed all political and religious lines. People needed help, and there were people there to help. As in the hospitals of the Middle Ages, a foundation of medicine is the virtue of charity.

I saw that spirit of charity—of being made to give—in Bangladesh, where I ended up after meeting Dr. Herbert Coddington. He had been a missionary to Korea and had reached retirement age, but wasn't ready to retire. He decided to work in an area where there was need, and that was in Bangladesh as civil war erupted in the 1970s. I met him in Massachusetts later in his life. I remember him saying that I didn't look like the type of person who would do medical relief work. He said I looked too much like someone looking for fun. After all, I had a sports car. I'm sure that when he invited me to work with him in Bangladesh, he never really thought I would take him up on it.

But I went to Bangladesh a number of times with him. He was an amazing person and I was very touched by his work. I worked with him in a poor area of the capital, Dhaka. The clinic he built was right in front of the city dump. As I remember, it was supported by a gentleman from North Carolina. Dr. Coddington always used to say, "Pray for Mr. Scott because Mr. Scott is close to one hundred years old. Pray for his health." Mr. Scott turned out to be financing the clinic at about $50,000 USD a year, which basically paid the staff and clinic costs because Dr. Coddington never took any money for himself.

The staff certainly earned their pay. We would see maybe fifty or sixty patients a day in this poor little clinic that was just put together with a plastic and steel roof. We would see people with typhoid, malaria, tuberculosis. Dr. Coddington himself never stopped, and those who couldn't afford to pay were given free care. This was in the 1980s, and the cost for full care, including medications, for everything from tuberculosis to typhoid fever or malaria couldn't have been more than twenty or twenty-five cents. However, some of our patients couldn't afford even that. For those patients who couldn't afford to pay, Dr. Coddington would refer them to the "poor fund," which basically meant Dr. Coddington would pay from his own pocket.

I also worked at Malumghat Hospital in Chittagong, Bangladesh. It was started by a man named Dr. Olsen in 1966. I stayed for about three months. Initially, I was there to fill in for other doctors when they went on temporary leave for vacation.

Suddenly, I was thrown into a situation where everybody left, and I was placed in charge of surgical and medical services.

I have had very minimal surgical training other than through my internship. At that time, because my Christian faith had started to grow, I began seeing how God provided for me in situations where I needed to rise to the challenge in front of me. And here was a challenge indeed.

The surgeon left on a well-deserved vacation—something he hadn't done in years—and I was suddenly faced with being solely responsible for surgical cases. Other than having held retractors and done some skin surgery, I had no surgical experience at all. If I wasn't able to handle it, we would need to transfer patients with surgical emergencies to another hospital in Chittagong, which was at least a three-hour ride. There was the problem of transport, and the great possibility that poor patients would not have gone, either because of their fragile medical condition or their inability to pay for the costs associated with transport.

And then, as if out of nowhere, came a tall woman literally riding a Harley-Davidson. It was like something out of a book or movie. Her name was Zoe, which in the Bible means "life" and was adopted by Hellenized Jews as a cognate of Eve or first woman.

Zoe came in and said with her British accent, "I'm just driving through. Do you need any help with surgery?" I said, "Well, as a matter of fact, we do need a surgeon." I remember how tall she stood over me. Years later I would wonder out loud to my kids whether, with a coincidence like that, she was actually an angel.

We had a whole series of kids coming in with appendicitis, and she showed me how to do an appendectomy. She would say, "You're making such a bloody mess." Somehow, I got through it and learned from her how to do an appendectomy.

My attitude became "Oh, okay, let it happen." Whether Zoe was an angel or not, I don't know. But she was one of many amazing people I met who just wanted to help. Whether from a sense of duty or responsibility or a desire to serve, she came out of the middle of nowhere and helped me and so many young patients.

Not everyone rode up on a Harley Davidson. Whenever we were worried about pneumonia, we would get x-rays. We had neither faxes nor internet. So, a fellow carrying an umbrella while riding a bicycle would come to my room in the rain during monsoon season. He'd bring the x-rays so I could look at them. We felt pretty advanced just having x-rays to help confirm a diagnosis of pneumonia.

Malumghat is close to the border of Burma, and lots of very poor hill people would come for help. I often felt sorry for them. Yet there was a drive for life wherever I went, whatever the culture. I remember just seeing people coming from long distances, taking extreme risks for their children to bring them for wherever care they could—because life is valuable, regardless of the culture.

I saw the same thing when I worked as a medical director in the Ivory Coast during the early 1990s. I remember one woman who brought her son about one hundred miles to get medical care in the clinic where I was working in a village called Korhogo. I made the diagnosis of appendicitis, and as I was driving her and her son to the hospital, because we couldn't operate at the clinic, she said, "Please save my son; this is my last son."

She had already lost several of her children. She had no money. We had worked out a way to ensure that everybody who needed care would get care. The son survived. He got through the surgery. We made arrangements with a surgeon from Egypt at the local hospital. Normally, the local hospital insisted everybody pay, but we worked an arrangement for shared payment. The Egyptian surgeon provided free care without charging. It was real cooperation with everybody helping and working together for the common good.

It wasn't all miracles and angels on motorcycles by any means. Much of it was sad, and the month I spent in Somalia during the civil war in the 1990s was extremely dangerous. There was an area known as Bermuda because if you went there, supposedly it was like the Bermuda Triangle: You probably would never come out alive. There were gangs that would simply kill you for whatever equipment they could take it to sell. People were in very dire circumstances, and desperately seeking help.

What strikes me now is how badly they wanted to get well because the idea of wanting to die was totally foreign to them. Did they value life less because they were in a war zone? No, they valued life more. It's here in the West, where we've got such comfort, that we can't see the value of life.

We are the ones who don't put value on life. Even governments have bought into this. In our public healthcare systems, we're willing to take the life of someone who is elderly. We're also willing to abort unborn babies. We have 101 reasons why those elderly people and those babies are inconvenient. We will invoke death because people want to choose it. We don't stop to ask ourselves, "Is it a real choice; are people even aware of what they're doing?"

The Christian faith I learned as a child, even though I set it aside for a period of my life, taught me deep down the falseness of choosing to treat life like a disposable inconvenience. As a Boy Scout I learned to do my best, to be prepared, but I also gained the practical skill of first aid to help someone who was injured, who needed help. I learned that being made to live means we are made to give.

Seeing that play out across cultures shows me there is eternity in each person's heart. There's a life force that God has given us.

We cannot deny it, no matter how sophisticated we think we are, because it goes against the very nature of the human spirit. The Nazis tried to deny it in the 1930s and 1940s. They tried to say that only certain lives were worthy. That kind of thinking brought their leadership cadre to Nuremberg, and their dictator to suicide in an underground bunker.

Compare that to what I experienced in Haiti in 1990, working on a ward in the Hospital of Light where there were a lot of AIDS patients. We knew what AIDS was, but we didn't have any treatment for it. One patient was having trouble breathing this particular day, and I started to help him. The patient had TB, too, and multiple other diseases.

Then, one of the other patients, who was also quite sick with AIDS, stepped in to relieve me, and a young woman started to help, too. There were no antivirals for AIDS. As doctors, we were just treating the complications: the pneumonias, the diarrheas. We were hydrating patients, comforting them. We couldn't treat the underlying disease. But I will never forget the image of those people trying to help each other.

The young woman who came to help was so sick—she was wasting away. Yet she was running here, and running there, and helping another patient. It was terrible for all of those patients—it was really a death ward. But we didn't inject them. We didn't kill them. We didn't say, "Oh, your life is hopeless. We're going to give up on you. We're going to kill you." And they were helping each other in that dying ward.

The Romans and the Nazis, millennia apart, came to see suicide, even assisted suicide as an authentic and legitimate end to human life. Although we differ radically from both those cultures in crucially important ways, seventy-five years after Nuremberg we have come to accept their underlying utilitarian view of life's purpose and value. By legalizing euthanasia and assisted suicide, we agree that human beings are made to be disposed of, not made to live.

What I saw in Haiti, and in so many other countries where I worked, refutes such utilitarianism, and demonstrates the irrefutable truth of Jesus' parable of the Good Samaritan. What I have witnessed first-hand over decades of travel as a doctor is that the human drive is not to kill each other. It is to help each other. That is how we are called, how we are made—to live.

Chapter 8
Choosing Life

As a young doctor just starting out, I accompanied a young woman to an abortion clinic in the U.S. It was all very legal and safe. From the perspective of the state, society, and even prevailing medical ethics, it was all very much above board and proper.

Yet it was time of intense moral quandary for me. I was deeply uncomfortable because, as a doctor, I knew that was a child. A baby. A real baby. It meant taking a life. At the same time, the world said it was her choice to make, and given the options in front of her, it was the choice she chose.

I feel the loss even now. Not a horrible loss of paralyzing depressing gloom or regret—I don't think regrets have to be like that. I think they can be about how we might have changed the situation; what would we have done today now that we know more about life; what if we had said the word, phrase, or sentence that might have changed everything? In other words, real regret for a lost life that I can't bring back. In reality, that life was irredeemably lost the minute the "choice" was made, and the conviction took hold that it was the only available choice, that there was no turning back.

Would it have been possible to just refuse to accompany her through that choice? Maybe, but I did not. As so often happens when we try to fix a problem, we create another one. In that curious way we have as humans, doing what I felt was right created for me the lifelong problem of an indelible memory about participating in what I knew in my heart was wrong.

In all such moral turmoil and conundrums, sooner or later we come face to face with Jesus' eternal question: Who are we to judge? In the euthanasia, assisted suicide, MAiD mentality, the query itself is justification for moral abandonment to the utilitarian ethos of the Romans, the Nazis, and other political or cultural systems that insist that effectiveness, functionality, whether something "works" to its intended end, are the only ground for judgement. The euthanasia mindset epitomizes such utility perfectly by conforming exactly to the old ironic saying: "The procedure was a great success. But the patient died."

Jesus wasn't saying, though, that we must abandon judgement. Nor does the Bible, anywhere, oblige us to throw up our hands in the face of necessary judgement and just go with what looks like the easiest one. In both Testaments, we are constantly exhorted to make sure our choices come from right places and right attitudes: from charity, not vanity; from service, not self-indulgence; from obedience to God, not from coveting the whole world while losing our souls; finally and above all, from not disturbing ourselves over the speck in our neighbour's eye when we yet have a log in our own.

In the narrative of the woman taken in adultery, Jesus challenges those who are without sin to cast the first stone. St. Paul serves up the reminder that all have sinned and fall short of the glory of God. Both are essential cautionary distinctions between onerous judgements and slothful judgementalism. But contemporary thinking, which is vividly on display when it comes to euthanasia, assisted suicide, and MAiD, tends to compress judgement and judgementalism into a single sloppy amorphous wad and then abandon even the human capacity to judge right from wrong, moral from immoral. Simply put, it's OK to judge right from wrong, but it's not OK to be judgemental.

As I deepened in medical experience, and began returning truly to my Christian faith, I saw such abandonment not as progress but as a draining away of courage within society as a whole. By courage, I don't mean to imply some kind of Rambo warrior mentality with bandoliers of bullets across our chests. I mean it in the Biblical sense that encourages us to go on toward God even in the face of the worst difficulties, that encourages us not to give in to the easy, utilitarian solution. I mean it in the way Jesus says to His disciples throughout the Gospels: *"Be not afraid"* (for example, see Mark 5:36, Mark 6:50, or John 14:27).

Part of our general failure of courage is seeing happiness as the goal of all things. We don't mean, as the Greeks did, happiness as balance. We mean the opposite. We mean giddiness; we mean unceasing stimulation and amusement. We mean what the thinker Neil Postman described in the title of a 1985 book as "amusing ourselves to death."[81] We mean eternal euphoria, which is so perfectly apropos in any discussion of euthanasia.

Even worse, though, is the paradox that our endless pursuit of happiness as amusement unto death has led to us living very isolated lives. People are disconnected from community, from one another, whether it's a church community, or mealtime, or families. Everyone is very far off in their own little world.

We have this idea that we must be self-sufficient. If we're not self-sufficient, then it's not worth going on. The argument is, well, if I lose my autonomy, then I'm better off dead. No! We're

---

[81] Neil Postman, *Amusing Ourselves to Death: Public Discourse in the Age of Show Business* (New York: Viking Penguin, 1985).

better off in community. We depend on each other. We need to help each other. That's why we strive for healthcare for all. In Canada, we have a universal system of healthcare, which is by no means perfect. Medicines and some services are provided by a combination of private and public coverage. In the United States, there is a combination of private and public healthcare. Europe has a combination of various systems. But the goal is to ensure access to healthcare for all. That's why we've structured society to let us flourish in the reality that human beings are made to give as well as to live.

Finishing on top of the hill all alone is, to me, a losing proposition. If we go up the hill together, then we're winners. If we help each other and pull each other up the hill, then we're winners, but not alone. I think the society of autonomy and self-direction as the greatest good is wrong. The greatest virtue is helping one another. It's loving our neighbour as ourselves.

In its state of dying courage, of pursuing euphoria all the way to the isolation of death, contemporary society recycles the old judgementalism that if you can't contribute to society, then your life has no quality. If you are weak, how can you bear the burdens of life? In fact, you, in your weakened state, are the burden that must be put down—in both senses of that phrase. And in such a society, do we seriously believe there is such a thing as informed consent?

A study of those who signed up for assisted suicide in Oregon showed pain and suffering to be one of the least cited reasons for making that choice, according to the families. Far more common were loss of autonomy, loss of self-control, feelings of being a burden, and the big one—fear of being alone. Almost nothing about pain and suffering. The euthanasia and assisted suicide mindset has been marketed by attacking people's failing courage and preying on their fear that they will end their lives as a worthless human burden or, worse, alone. It is the result of fearmongering that tells people, "You're going to have a horrible, terrible quality of life if you don't end your life. But it's your choice." Stahle describes this process as the "dehumanization of the person": "The action of euthanasia and assisted suicide is justified by claiming that the patient's quality of life is so low that death is a better alternative."[82]

By accompanying someone through an abortion as a young doctor, I discovered that choices do not cease to exist just because we've made them. They can linger on in our own lives, and in the lives of others, even after a life itself is lost. Choice, then, isn't always a positive good, despite what the proponents of abortion and end-of-life termination insist. In the context of euthanasia, assisted suicide, and MAiD, choice is not always the patient's decision made alone in a bubble.

One of the things I have become increasingly aware of—in fact, I've had it impressed on me very aggressively at times—is the way medical resources are now considered choices rather than necessities. In a way that wasn't so when I began my medical career; we are now constantly told that the hospital, the clinic, the healthcare system, the state, doesn't have an endless amount of resources. So, in turn, we are told to focus on taking care of those who are survivable, which borrows from the language of disaster and triage. In triage, those who are more likely to survive get the resources. Those deemed less likely are to be left aside.

Of course, it's an outrageously false comparison. It's not the same thing at all. In day-to-day medicine, we do have the resources. It's the willingness to make them available that's at issue. It's not like a local hospital has multiple ambulances full of plane crash victims arriving at its doors on a daily or even weekly basis.

---

[82] Fabian Stahle, "Moral Disengagement—Mechanisms Propelling the Euthanasia/PAS Movement," *Journal of Ethics in Mental Health*, 10 (2017): 1–15.

Even when there's a disaster, we don't kill people whom we triage because they're less likely to survive. If they've survived, they will get the care. With end-of-life termination, however, the disaster-triage-resource management model is used to justify killing patients strictly to save the healthcare system money. This goes against all ethical models of all care. It is a model of uncaring.

When a person has reached the point where we don't see them getting better, it doesn't mean they *won't* get better. What's happening now is no guarantee of what will happen tomorrow or next week. Even when the person has said, "I don't want any acute care," that doesn't mean we don't still give comfort care: washing, bathing, providing fluids. You absolutely have to provide all those things.

The reality is that patients who get good quality pain control actually live longer. The concept of double effect—that if you increase the pain medication to control the pain then you eventually reach a dose that will actually kill the patient—has been proven not to be the case. There is no such thing as double effect. As long as you dose the pain medication according to the pain, you won't end the patient's life.

Pain treatment for many chronic diseases is improving, and it will continue to improve if research funding is made a priority. In the Western World, there are many chronic diseases of aging including heart disease, cancer, kidney and lung disease. There also needs to be more research and investment in pediatric care, including pediatric cancer care. The recent announcement by the President of the United States in his State of the Union address to fund pediatric cancer with $500 million over the next ten years is a step in the right direction.[83] Nevertheless, much more needs to be done.

---

[83] "Remarks by President Trump in State of the Union Address," Feb. 5, 2019 (https://www.whitehouse.gov/briefings-statements/remarks-president-trump-state-union-address-2/).

Recently, the United States has also opened up innovative treatments for incurable diseases that heretofore required FDA approval, which delayed promising new treatments. According to the BBC:

President Donald Trump has signed a bill giving terminally ill patients the right to try experimental treatments not approved by the government....

"... We never give up, right?" Mr Trump said to patients and their families during a bill signing ceremony at the White House....

After signing the bill, Mr Trump handed his pen to nine-year-old Jordan McLinn, who has been diagnosed with a form of terminal muscular dystrophy.

Jordan, who the bill is named for, has been accepted into a clinical program in Chicago where he has been receiving weekly infusions.

He and his mother, Laura, had travelled from Indianapolis for the White House event.[84]

Obviously, if people don't want a particular treatment, we don't force it on them. But that is very different from intentionally killing a person. When Hippocrates came up with his tenets for healthcare 2500 years ago, there were physicians who would kill people. If you had an enemy, you could pay a physician to kill them. It is why people were afraid to go to a physician: they didn't know if he was going to kill them. Today, it's much the same thing. You don't know who they're going to kill. We've gone backwards.

We think choice is a good in itself. At the same time, our supposed end-of-life choice is conditioned in ways we can't imagine

---

[84] "Trump Signs Right to Try Act for Terminally Ill Patients," *BBC.com*, May 30, 2018 (https://www.bbc.com/news/world-us-canada-44305998).

by people whose highest good is the triage-style management of medical resources bought and paid for through our tax dollars. Here is another psychological mechanism that leads to moral disengagement.

> When using the catchphrase "personal choice", the responsibility is transferred to the patient (displacement of responsibility). It is the patient's own decision, they say, but the patient may often, even subtly and unconsciously, be guided in one direction or the other by doctors and relatives. In addition, legalization in itself implies pressure, since society thereby proclaims that suicide is a recommended measure in certain situations.[85]

Who is the real enemy of choice, of good medicine, of being made to live here?

Which brings us full circle to the birth of the little girl whose words created the title of this book. Although I had long been on a path of change as a Christian, a doctor, a father, a husband, and many other roles, something changed in me profoundly because of what I went through with my family around Jessica's birth. It gave me a new hope, a new meaning for life, and the courage to join those battling against euthanasia, assisted suicide, and MAiD.

If I had followed the advice of my colleagues, all that would have been loss. I do not, in any way, mean that as a disparagement of them in their ethics or medical professionalism. I know they were acting the way the current spirit of death obliges them to act—that is, as modern-day secular humanists. They were acting as we have all been taught to act: giving priority to guaranteed good outcomes, and minimizing risk—even a risk on life.

---

[85] Fabian Stahle, "Moral Disengagement—Mechanisms Propelling the Euthanasia/PAS Movement," *Journal of Ethics in Mental Health*, 10 (2017): 1–15.

The older approach is that if you don't take a risk on life, you're going to miss the joys life has to offer. There is pain and there is joy. They are part of a continuum. They come together. You can't get one without the other. If you don't try, you will live a very sterile life.

It's like living on the hundredth floor of a modern downtown high-rise. There's a beautiful view that lets you see the whole city landscape. There's filtered air. You can't open your windows. Very bare, minimalist furniture. Frequently, you live alone, and you don't really get to know your neighbours. You have all your basic needs met. But you spend your time communicating by cell phone or text or Instagram.

Real life on the ground involves risks that we live every day. And the risk with Jessica was that we weren't going to have a good outcome. But we took the risk because we believed that this was a life and we could not—even for our own benefit, even though it might become inconvenient—do anything less than everything for her. We erred on the side of life with all there is that comes with it.

By giving, we were given back infinite treasure. We made sacrifices, but they were a pittance compared to the richness returned. Even when we were in intensive care, we would meet with other families in the family room at the old Montreal Children's Hospital. They, too, all had amazing stories of challenges. They were all holding onto the hope of life for their child, a future for their child. We shared the struggles we were having. We were amazed at their courage and strength, and when they heard our story, they were inspired by our courage and strength.

None of it was planned. They didn't set up the family room expressly so we could meet these other families. It was there, basically, so we could warm up whatever food we had and eat and talk together as a couple. I learned from that when you struggle through the difficulties, as you go day to day not knowing the future, it draws you closer as a couple, it draws you closer to other people who are going through struggles, and it makes you appreciate the gift of life given to each of us that much more.

We would never have learned all those things without going through the experience, the struggle. I do know we would have lost huge pieces of our souls—big chunks of our hearts—because Jessica has provided us with tremendous joy. She is the funniest. She is very strong-willed. And with her, my son tends to be much gentler, much kinder. John-Anthony sometimes finds it hard to take an "older brother stance" with her because she's such a strong character. It comes from her struggle to survive. And I try to always share that with the family. It's good for him, too. Gentleness, kindness isn't weakness. And he, too, is certainly a strong young man.

I have probably spoiled Jessica more than Eliana or John-Anthony. The older two accuse me of doing it. She insisted on getting a dog, so I bought her a little dog. The others had pleaded for one for many years, but it was Jessica's plea that really touched my heart.

I'm just amazed every day when I see her, and her older siblings are too. We all appreciate her so much because of that spirit, that strong free spirit to live that she has.

When she puts her mind to something, she just plows ahead. We've seen that in every aspect—whether it's her music or her schooling, when she decides she's going to do something, she does it. We can't imagine a life without Jessica. Yet we were told, in different ways, that we would be better off doing just that.

When I was going through medical school, we studied embryogenesis. We looked at the development of the embryo, the fetus. But it was all very mechanical: when the heart develops, when the limbs form, when the brain forms. But there was no real emotion or soul. Obviously, we talked about flesh on the bones, but that was more of a physical flesh on bones—it didn't have real meaning.

With the pregnancy of our first daughter, Eliana, we were so overjoyed, and then my wife had some spotting. They called us to come down to the Royal Victoria Hospital, and scheduled an ultrasound. And Eliana was about six weeks old on that ultrasound. We could see a little beating heart. It was the size of a bean, and that's exactly what the ultrasonographer said: "A little bean." So, we called her Little Bean.

I was amazed. You know, you go back, you read your medical textbooks and they confirm that, yes, the heart starts beating at five or six weeks. But this was our daughter! She wasn't just a little picture in a book. She was a real living human being. It became reality.

Then when Jessica was about twenty weeks, they told us to look at our options. I immediately said "no," but what really came to my inner soul was what had happened many years earlier when I was a young doctor accompanying that young woman to the abortion clinic. I started remembering my realization that once you've made the decision, you can't go back. You can't bring back something that is lost.

I have older patients who will share with me the regrets of having lost a child that way. I don't bring it up at first—they do. They bring up their history on their own. They will talk about it if they're depressed, or having regrets, or faced with some difficulty in life. I'll ask, "What is it you regret? What are your thoughts?" And then I will share my story in a way that shows there's a future and a hope, that there is a forgiving God.

It's kind of like a twelve-step program: God forgives, and if there are people you've hurt, that you can make amends to, then make those amends. Take an inventory of your life. My patients are sometimes overwhelmed with anxiety and fear for the future.

I suggest they take an inventory of their lives. I let them know they're not alone. If there are things they can change, try to change them. If there are things they can't, leave them to God.

The message I want you to take away is to stand strong. Be courageous. Do not fear. It's hard for us to rely on our own strength. But we can call out to God, whom I understand as a loving, caring God—represented through Jesus Christ, whom I think the faithful of all religions will agree was one of the most amazing people ever to walk this earth

We all want to have control of our lives. That's a normal human trait. We want to control bad situations, and we want to be able to manage things. For physicians, one of our jobs is to try to help people who are faced with illness, some of them life-threatening. The solution isn't to end the process prematurely, whether through abortion or medical termination. It's to be there. It's to support.

That's not prescribing passive acceptance. It's not saying, "Oh, I'll just cross my arms and do nothing." But by ending a person's life, you're doing damage—perhaps the most damage possible—even through you may not know what the final outcome will be. Things *can* turn around.

I think of my patient Mona, who was told by a doctor that her life was going to end very shortly with lung disease. I think of Alexander, who mistakenly thought he had lung cancer. If they had both chosen rapid solutions to end their situation because it was causing them psychological or physical suffering at the time, they would have lost life, just as we would have lost Jessica had we gone down that recommended path.

Far more harm than good would have been done. Yet one thing would have been temporarily satisfied: our social addiction to control. Euthanasia and assisted suicide have become another societal addiction, just like all the others for which there are now twelve-step programs, to control situations that people feel desperate about.

When we hear proponents for euthanasia and assisted suicide talk about the autonomy of the individual, they invariably talk about giving control to the individual. But what they call control for the individual actually requires the individual's self-destruction. It requires destroying the lives of those who are allegedly exercising their autonomy and control. This is the problem for all addictions.

With all addictions, we want to have a sense of being able to manipulate and control outcomes. And we don't. As a physician, I move a person toward health, toward healthy living, toward a good outcome. But I don't know the outcomes, and I can't guarantee the outcomes. I can say we will try. If, as a physician, I claim to know with perfect certainty what the outcomes will be for my patient, I'm playing God—and when you try to play God, you're playing Russian roulette. You will get the worst of all imaginable outcomes. You will have absolutely zero control.

It is very difficult for many who come from the sciences to admit that life is a big unknown. For a lot of doctors, whose business is life, it can be a major and difficult exercise in humility. Yet it's true. Life is a big unknown.

We have some understanding of physiology, of biochemistry, of neurology and all the different -ologies that we study in medicine. Pathology. Pulmonology. Cardiology. We know things about how medication works. We know a bit about how the body ages. Even the best scientists will tell you we still know relatively little about the human brain. We are far, far from knowing everything, and we certainly don't know outcomes.

What we do know about is caring and loving, even though that is limited. We can only care as much as we allow ourselves to care. We only love as much as we allow ourselves to love. If we end a life, we can no longer care for that person. They become a memory, but we can't actively care. How, by ending a life, do we show we truly care for the person? At best, it's a very truncated, low-cost kind of caring. We'll throw a party for you and hold your hand as they give you the injection. Is that true caring?

People have challenged me and said, "What do you mean? I cared." You cared up to a point—as long as the person was there. But after that? I had a woman come to see me recently whose mother died at ninety-three. She had moved into her house. She cared for her mom the last ten years of her life as she dwindled. She was there as her mom passed away. That is caring. That is sacrificial caring.

Her sister, she said, would call occasionally, but never visited. My patient came to my office because she was very stressed. The stress occurred afterward when they sold the house. Her sister wanted her part of the inheritance, so the one who sacrificed had to move out.

But the one who stayed said to me: "I don't regret a moment. I have to move out. I have to find another place, somewhere smaller. But I don't regret the ten years, because I spent them caring for my mom."

Her mom had requested to never be put into a nursing home. She said it would be the end of her. And the daughter respected her mother's desire right to the end. That, to me, is a witness of powerful love and caring.

Nevertheless, there are situations where family members are unable to care for loved ones at home. In some cases, this is because homecare systems are lacking. Nevertheless, as a caring society we must decide to provide for those needs. In other cases, the decision is made to care for people in facilities when family members cannot provide the care because the healthcare needs overwhelm the caregiver's capacities, either financially, temporally, or physically. But this does not obviate our need to visit, be present with, and participate in caring and loving—even if that takes the form of helping to prepare and accompanying during mealtime.

Now, people who are in favour of euthanasia and assisted suicide will say, "But I respect the desire of the person to die." The difference is that to end a person's life, you are bringing their life to an end, even if that person asks you to please end it. This is intentional killing.

You must accompany the person until that life ceases to exist. Our responsibility is to accompany—that is, to care for—each fellow human being. Not just in a professional capacity as physicians, but as a society. As children. As brothers and sisters. As parents, just like we were faced to with the choice to end the life of our new daughter but instead said, "No. We will always say 'yes' to life. And Jessica Saba is made to live."

AFTERWORD

As I alluded to early in the book, the battle against euthanasia has been exhausting, both physically and financially. To fight against it is to grapple with one of the truly dark forces of our day, however good and decent and well-intentioned the proponents of it may be. Just as this book was being completed, for example, yet another wave of blackness washed over us with news that Quebec's Superior Court had struck down the restrictions that limited MAiD to terminally ill patients under both federal and Quebec legislation.

Unfortunately, Justice Christine Baudouin's mid-September 2019 ruling struck down the "reasonably foreseeable" provision of the legislation that provided at least some measure of restraint. The ruling was suspended for six months to allow legislators to make the necessary legislative amendments, but Justice Baudouin permitted the two people who brought the constitutional challenge, Jean Truchon and Nicole Gladu, to receive MAiD anyway.

Justice Baudouin accepted as sufficient Mr. Truchon's testimony that because of his cerebral palsy, "He can no longer live on his own…. He says he has been dead since 2012."[86] Of course, he has been very much alive—enough to undertake challenges to laws that came into existence well after the claimed date of his death. Also, the judge didn't consider the possibility that Mr. Truchon might have chosen to live and not seek euthanasia if he'd been given the means to live at home independently rather than being institutionalized.

As for the seventy-three-year-old Ms. Gladu, who has lived with polio for sixty-nine years, the court ruled she was a "prisoner of her body and illness" despite her being perfectly free to fight the case. It did not take long for the slippery slope to get even more slippery and steep. According to the Canadian Press, at a press conference on January 21, 2020, Quebec's Health Minister was reported to plan to extend MAiD to "people with mental health issues who aren't responding to treatment."[87] While the Minister seemed to sidestep mere days later, stating that a consultation process would take place prior to any final decision about extending euthanasia to depressed people, it appears that it is only a matter of time before such legislation is proposed.[88]

With such troubled, dangerous thinking dominating our courts, our legislatures, our media, and to an extent even some of our churches, it's no wonder I have seen many people initially engage in the fight against it, and then move on to other issues simply because of the spiritual toll it takes. Those who've stayed—

---

[86] Tu Thanh Ha & Kelly Grant, "Quebec Court Strikes Down Restriction to Medically Assisted Dying Law, Calls It Unconstitutional," *Globe and Mail*, Sept. 12, 2019 (https://www.theglobeandmail.com/life/health-and-fitness/article-quebec-court-strikes-down-parts-of-laws-on-medically-assisted-death/).

[87] Sidhartha Banerjee, "Quebec to Expand Assisted Death to Mentally Ill, but Few Expected to Qualify," *660 News*, January 22, 2020 (https://www.660citynews.com/2020/01/22/quebec-to-expand-assisted-death-to-mentally-ill-but-few-expected-to-qualify/).

[88] Lia Levesque, "Quebec to Seek Consensus on Offering Medical Aid in Dying to Mentally Ill," *CTV News*, January 27, 2020 (https://montreal.ctvnews.ca/quebec-to-seek-consensus-on-offering-medical-aid-in-dying-to-mentally-ill-1.4784859).

and those who've left—are truly amazing people, and I am privileged to have met them on this road.

I am an optimist by nature. I do not personally believe many genuine pessimists make it into, much less through, medical school. Fewer pessimists still would stick with a medical practice for many years.

At one point in the struggle, however, I began talking to my wife Marisa about my own options. Because of my mother's American birth, I remain a U.S. citizen. I could take the parachute, put the family in the car, fill the moving van, and go to a non-euthanasia, non-assisted suicide state like Kentucky. Why Kentucky? Why not join an Amish community or enter a monastery?

It took a while to get Marisa to walk through the prospective plan with me. Part of the reason is my ingrained habit of suddenly giving her my latest brilliant insight about some situation such as, well, moving to Kentucky while we're in the middle of her trying to rush to get to an appointment.

Her standard response is, "Not right now."

And I wheedle a bit and say, "But honey, I think I've got a solution."

And she will say, "I've got to get the kids to the dentist. And a nuclear bomb's about to hit us, so we need to hit the basement after we get back from the dentist but before the tornado touches down this afternoon. So not right now, Paul."

Finally, though, in the midst of the family rush, we talked about moving. Marisa said one of the most amazing things she's said to me in sixteen years of marriage. She said, "Now you can talk." So I told her my brilliant idea of us moving to Kentucky. I like Kentucky. People I've met from Kentucky are amazing. But I got the feeling she wasn't as keen on Kentucky as I was. Not because it was Kentucky, but for some entirely un-Kentucky-related reason.

"Paul," she said, "what impact are you going to have on the lives of these people that you've touched over all these years if you're in Kentucky? If you think it will make a statement, all they'll know is that you ran away. That's exactly what it will appear to be. And that's exactly what it'll be. Are you somebody who runs away?"

The only vocalized answer for a boy born and raised in Lachine, Quebec whose grandparents were from Lebanon was, of course, "No."

In my head, though, I was doing a little happy dance that I'd married her—not because she was smart enough to have married me, but because she knows so much that I will never know.

Then I remembered hearing someone once say to make an impact on people's lives it's better to be in Hell's backyard than at Heaven's gates. Right now, in Canada and Quebec, that's where I live, and it's where I need to stay and fight.

Beyond staying to fight as an individual, I am committed to moving others to recognize the medical travesty and spiritual darkness that euthanasia, assisted suicide, and MAiD present us with. One of the delights of preparing this book has been to see the way that spirit has moved my own family, including my eldest daughter, Eliana. She took on the task of researching the vital need to direct our efforts toward radically improved treatment, especially of childhood diseases, rather than termination. Here are her findings and her call to action in the form of a very pointed question:

Tracy is a woman in her forties who suffers from muscular dystrophy. I first met her before Christmas of 2017. She was living in a special unit for patients with chronic neurological and life-threatening disorders. She has lived with this neurological disorder all her life. She is confined to a wheelchair. She can breathe on her own but needs breathing support at night. Her brother has the same disorder.

They live in two adjacent rooms in the unit. Their mother is a retired social worker who visits every day to heat up special meals and to encourage and support her children. What struck me about Tracy is her beautiful and radiant smile. She is always happy, despite everything she has been through. Unfortunately there is no successful treatment for her neurological disorder.

People with neurological disorders are generally presented in the media in a negative light. In society they are often shunned, mocked, and avoided. My dad has worked on a ward with people with neurological disorders because he believes that every life is valuable. He has also been fighting euthanasia and assisted suicide for as long as I can remember. He believes that all of these neurological diseases could be cured if we invested enough into research.

I decided to research some of these neurological disorders. I have listed the top seven most common neurological diseases globally along with their clinical presentation, known treatments, and future research possibilities.

1. DEMENTIA

Dementia is a disease that affects a person's memory, preventing them from carrying out activities of daily living. The most common form of dementia is Alzheimer's, which makes up approximately 65% of cases. According to the World Health Organization, "Almost 9.9 million people develop dementia each year… Dementia currently affects approximately 50 million people worldwide; a number that is projected to grow to 82 million by 2030 and 152 million by 2050. It is the second largest cause of disability for individuals aged 70 years and older, and the seventh leading cause of death. Dementia imposes an estimated economic cost of approximately US$ 818 billion per year globally. This is equivalent to 1.1% of global gross domestic product."[89]

The World Health Organization has targeted a seven-step action plan to combat the effects of dementia worldwide, including the need for more awareness and research. Presently, there is no effective medical treatment to prevent and cure this disease.

2. PARKINSON'S

Parkinson's disease is the second most common neurodegenerative disease behind Alzheimer's. It affects one in one hundred people after the age of sixty. It is characterized by motor symptoms including rigidity, tremors, speech impairment, difficulty swallowing, and frequent falls. It is chronic and progressive and is often diagnosed after sixty. However, five percent of patients become symptomatic before that age. It is a tremendous burden on families and their caregivers, causing people to lose their jobs and source of income. Sixty thousand people are diagnosed with Parkinson's disease each year in the United States, with one million people presently affected. The main state of treatment has been drug therapy including dopaminergic drugs. There are new treatments including deep-brain stimulation, but there is no definitive cure.[90]

---

[89] *Towards a Dementia Plan: A WHO Guide* (Geneva: World Health Organization, 2018) (https://apps.who.int/iris/bitstream/handle/10665/272642/9789241514132-eng.pdf?ua=1).

[90] Emily Downward & Jessica Johns Pool, "How Common Is Parkinson's Disease?," *Parkinsonsdisease.net,* September 2019 (https://parkinsonsdisease.net/basics/statistics/).

3. MULTIPLE SCLEROSIS (MS)

During my time visiting some of the patients where my dad worked, I met a young neuroscientist who had developed multiple sclerosis in her twenties. She was in a wheelchair and needed medications to help alleviate her muscle spasms and pain. Despite undergoing treatments, she had not been cured, and required constant care for her basic needs. Her husband, who also has MS, lived in the adjacent room. I enjoyed talking to Patricia,[91] who was hopeful that a cure would be discovered.

Multiple sclerosis affects over 2.5 million people worldwide.[92] It affects the central nervous system, and has many symptoms including blurred and loss of vision, poor coordination, weakness, memory loss, and even paralysis. It can affect young people like Patricia. It is believed to be an immune mediated disorder, but the cause is currently unknown. There are a number of drugs that modify the course of the disease, but there is no cure.

4. STROKE

I recently reviewed an online advanced life support course with my dad.[93] In the course, I learned about the early recognition of stroke. This rapid assessment tool is known as the Cincinnati Prehospital Stroke Scale (facial droop, arm drift, speech impairment). It is important to treat strokes rapidly with clot-busting drugs (thrombolysis) less than 4.5 hours after confirming the diagnosis by a CT scan.

Stroke is the third most common cause of death in industrialized countries. Most strokes are caused by the

---

[91] Name changed to protect patient confidentiality.

[92] National Multiple Sclerosis Society, "Multiple Sclerosis FAQs" ((https://www.nationalmssociety.org/What-is-MS/MS-FAQ-s)

[93] https://www.aclsmedicaltraining.com/acls-certification-online/.

blockage of blood flow to the brain, and are known as ischemic strokes. Smoking, diabetes, and obesity are preventable causes of strokes. Strokes are a major cause of disability, with one in three persons being severely disabled. It has been estimated that strokes account for about six percent of the total national health and social service expenditure in the United Kingdom. According to my calculations, if the United States spent the same percent on healthcare costs as the United Kingdom, it would be equal to approximately $194 billion in 2017. Thrombolysis is an effective treatment, but can only be given to around five percent of patients because of delays in seeking emergency care. Aspirin is also an effective and inexpensive treatment. If given immediately, it lowers the risk of early recurrent stroke and increases the chances of survival free of disability. Therefore, there must be more awareness of stroke, early diagnoses, lifestyle changes for prevention, and creation of more stroke units.[94]

5. MUSCULAR DYSTROPHY (MD)

According to Muscular Dystrophy Canada, there are over 150 neuromuscular diseases, which all weaken muscles. Amongst them is Muscular Dystrophy. Muscular Dystrophy is a rare disease caused by defects in a person's genes. Though it's rare, it can be extremely disabling in a young person's life. Principal symptoms include progressive muscle wasting, weakness, and loss of function. Common signs include poor balance with frequent falls, difficulty walking, limited range of

---

[94] *Neurological Disorders: Public Health Challenges* (Geneva: World Health Organization, 2006) (https://www.who.int/mental_health/neurology/neurological_disorders_report_web.pdf)

movement, and drooping eyelids. There is no cure, and more research has to be done.[95]

6. AMYOTROPHIC LATERAL SCLEROSIS (ALS)

My dad has described a number of patients who lived with ALS, also known as Lou Gehrig's disease. It was named after the famous New York Yankee baseball player who contracted the disease. It attacks the motor neurons, which leads to weakness and paralysis. Most people live an average of three to five years. There are no known cures, but there are promising new drugs that slow the progression of the disease. Around thirty thousand Americans are currently affected by this disease, with fifteen new cases diagnosed daily.[96]

7. MALNUTRITION ASSOCIATED NEUROLOGICAL DISORDERS

Malnutrition affects approximately eight hundred million children in the developing world, leading to a wide variety of neurological disorders that are preventable. The causes are: protein energy malnutrition, vitamin A deficiency (which can lead to blindness), lack of iodine (which can lead to stunted growth and mental retardation), and iron deficiency (which can lead to delayed mental development in children). The solution for malnutrition in the underdeveloped world is simple: more food, vitamins, and mineral supplementation.

WHERE DO WE GO FROM HERE?

The National Institute of Health (NIH) is the US government's research institute that supports research in

---

[95] http://www.muscle.ca/

[96] http://www.alsa.org/

finding cures for diseases. Their mission is "To enhance health, lengthen life, and reduce illness and disability." Their annual budget for 2019 was approximately 39.2 billion dollars. [97] Not only does the NIH help people live longer, healthier lives in the United States and the world, but it also creates jobs and stimulates the US economy. Increasing the budget of the NIH by about 5 billion dollars per year over the next ten years, will advance research and lead to better health outcomes. In addition, it will contribute to improving the US economy.

The Canadian Institutes of Health Research (CIHR) invests approximately one billion dollars per year in medical research. [98] An additional one hundred million dollars over the next ten years by the Canadian government will also promote research, improve health outcomes and stimulate the Canadian economy.

Since Canada and the United States are good neighbours and partners, they should work together to benefit health outcomes around the world.

Hopefully, the increased investment by both countries in healthcare research will set an example for other G20 countries, who can do the same. This will have a major impact on improving the world's health.

In the same manner, the G20 countries must invest in healthcare and research in the developing world. According to UNICEF, 5.4 million children under the age of five died in 2017.[99] A 2011 report states, "around 70% of these early child deaths are due to conditions

---

[97] National Institutes of Health, "What We Do" (https://www.nih.gov/about-nih/what-we-do)

[98] "Funding Overview," Canadian Institutes for Health Research (www.cihr-irsc.gc.ca/e/37788.html)

[99] "Under-Five Mortality," UNICEF (https://data.unicef.org/topic/child-survival/

that could be prevented or treated with access to simple, affordable interventions."[100] This would mean 3.5 million children's lives could be saved each year at minimal cost. Saving these lives has been estimated to cost about $4000 per child.[101] According to my calculation, this translates to approximately $14 billion per year to save 3.5 million children. Is this too much to ask for to save children's lives?

Throughout the book, I've wrestled with the paradox that confronts me daily as a doctor: We are given life knowing that ultimately we must die. But Eliana's question is really the one her coming generation will find itself facing. Is it too much to ask that we do all we can to save the lives of children, and all who are suffering, until the natural end? Can that possibly be too much to ask of us—God's people—who are made to live?

---

under-five-mortality)
[100] "Child Mortality," The Partnership for Maternal, Newborn & Child Health (2011) (https://www.who.int/pmnch/media/press_materials/fs/fs_mdg4_childmortality/en/)
[101] Sarah Boseley, "Investment in Child Health in World's Poorest Countries Saves 34m Lives," *The Guardian,* July 3, 2015.

Epilogue

Just as this book was being readied for printing, the COVID-19 pandemic hit the world and turned all of our lives upside down.

Hospitals were overwhelmed, and in certain countries people were unable to get access to medical care. There was a lack of ventilators and personal protective equipment. In certain countries, including Italy, people over sixty were denied access to life-saving ventilators. Triage systems were put into place to determine who would get medical care and who would be refused based on age and health risk factors.

In the United States and Canada, there were discussions and debates about implementing guidelines as to who would be given access to care. On May 21, 2020 the New England Journal of Medicine published a list of six recommendations on how to allocate medical resources during the COVID-19 pandemic.

These guidelines are based on the premise that there is a scarcity of medical resources, and are thus meant to "ensure that individual doctors are never tasked with deciding unaided which patients receive life-saving care and which do not. …(and) to alleviate physician burden and to ensure equal treatment."

The recommendations include prioritizing certain types of patients for curative treatments such as intensive care unit (ICU) beds and ventilators—namely, they "assign a higher priority for intensive care access to younger patients with severe illness than to elderly patients." Among the most important values is "the value of maximizing benefits" including "removing a patient from a ventilator or an ICU bed to provide it to others in need" even without the patient's consent.[102]

Not surprisingly, the Canadian Medical Association (CMA) quickly endorsed these recommendations in April 2020.[103] Similar to the CMA's framework, a COVID-19 triage protocol was drafted by Ontario Health and recommended "denying critical care to anyone with a less than 70% chance of survival, including anyone who scores as even mildly frail due to a progressive illness or condition."[104]

It is clear that these recommendations lead to discrimination based on age, pre-existing health conditions, and disability.

Some of the abandonment of ethical values was tragically demonstrated by the utter neglect of our seniors in nursing homes and the lack of protection of healthcare personnel. Seniors were left to die in abominable circumstances without their basic needs being met. They were forced to live in crowded facilities.

---

[102] E.J. Emanuel, G. Persad, R. Upshur, et al., "Fair Allocation of Scarce Medical Resources in the Time of Covid-19," *New England Journal of Medicine* 382 (May 21, 2020): 2049 – 2055 (https://www.nejm.org/doi/full/10.1056/NEJMsb2005114).

[103] Canadian Medical Assocation, "Framework for Ethical Decision Making During the Coronavirus Pandemic," April 2020 (https://policybase.cma.ca/en/viewer?file=%2fdocuments%2fPolicypdf%2fPD20-03.pdf).

[104] Brian Owens, "Should Triage Guidelines Be Revisited ahead of a Second Wave of COVID-19?," *CMAJ News,* June 3, 2020 (https://cmajnews.com/2020/06/03/covid-triage-1095876/).

In Quebec and some other provinces in Canada and some American states,[105, 106] COVID-positive patients were transferred back into nursing homes despite the risk—and consequence—of contaminating others still uninfected by COVID. Medical personnel were forced to work without basic protective equipment. Nursing homes became death houses. Despite some desperate last-minute efforts to reverse losses, everything was done "too little, too late."

One of the nurse's aides I cared for developed COVID-19 while caring for patients in a nursing home. She continued to care for her patients because "they were dehydrated and hungry and there was no one to give them something to drink or eat and clean them." Despite her weakened state, she was forced to work and finally called in sick because her "head hurt so much" that she "couldn't lift it off the bed." She was still off work at the time of writing.

This woman in her fifties has a number of chronic health issues and is of Black descent (which in itself is considered a negative risk factor for survival). Because of her multiple risk factors, she feared for her life if she ever got severely sick from COVID and needed hospitalization. She was afraid that she might face an uncertain future if "selected" as someone less likely to survive when healthcare resources were limited. Her fears are not unwarranted based on current guidelines and recommendations of medical resource allocation.

In contrast to the guidelines presented in the New England Journal and by the Canadian Medical Association, models

---

[105] Kelly Grant & Tu Thanh Ha, "How Shoring Up Hospitals for COVID-19 Contributed to Canada's Long-Term Care Crisis," *Globe and Mail*, May 21, 2020 (https://www.theglobeandmail.com/canada/article-how-shoring-up-hospitals-for-covid-19-contributed-to-canadas-long/).

[106] Olga Khazan, "The U.S. Is Repeating Its Deadliest Pandemic Mistake," *The Atlantic*, July 6, 2020 (https://www.theatlantic.com/health/archive/2020/07/us-repeating-deadliest-pandemic-mistake-nursing-home-deaths/613855/).

promoting improved public healthcare measures along with increased health system capacity demonstrate reductions or delays in health system collapse and resource depletion. The World Medical Association, which comprises over ten million physicians in 113 countries, urged governments worldwide to ensure personal protective equipment for personnel and a sufficient amount of beds in ICUs to treat all patients "without comprising ethical conditions." In October 2019, the WMA had reaffirmed its opposition to euthanasia and physician-assisted suicide, because there is no place in a caring society for devaluing any lives; rather, our priority should be saving all lives, including those afflicted by COVID-19.

Once again, the ethical debate raised during the COVID-19 pandemic clearly shows that we must develop a mindset of proactively caring for all people regardless of their age, health, socio-economic status, or disability during pandemics, catastrophes, revolutions, or wars. We must provide all the necessary resources to save life—because every life is valuable, and because we are made to live.

About the Author

Dr. Paul Saba is a physician who has studied, trained, and worked in Canada and the United States, and internationally in war-torn Lebanon and Somalia, in Bangladesh, Honduras, the Ivory Coast, and Haiti.

After completing medical school at McGill University in Montreal and a residency in Massachusetts, Dr. Saba worked in Massachusetts and later at Duke University Medical Center in North Carolina. While at Duke University Medical Center, Dr. Saba organized "Volunteering in the Developing World" conferences on children's health.

In the early 2000s, Dr. Saba worked in rural Quebec to keep emergency rooms open that might have closed because of a severe physician shortage.

In 2004 he began working at Lachine's St. Joseph Hospital, a community hospital that was at risk of closing, which he actively worked to save. His battle took him to the Quebec legislature, where he obtained a unanimous resolution to keep the hospital open. Today St. Joseph's is a full-service hospital that is part of the McGill University Health Centre and in the process of a major renovation project. For more than ten years, Dr. Saba has served as the hospital's President of the Council of Physicians. Today Lachine Hospital is one of Canada's top twenty hospitals.

Since 1998, Dr. Saba has actively worked to improve Quebec and Canada's publicly funded health care through the Coalition of Physicians for Social Justice, which he co-founded and presides over.

He has successfully fought for free medication for the disadvantaged, nutritional support for the elderly, and physical fitness for children.

In 2000, he examined, at no charge, patients from the Northeastern United States who bussed to Montreal to purchase less expensive lifesaving medicines in Canada.

He has made presentations opposing assisted suicide and euthanasia before state legislatures in New Hampshire, Connecticut, and New York, and before international forums in Rome, Italy; Reykjavik, Iceland; Santiago, Chile; and Tbilisi, Georgia.

Dr. Saba currently practises in Montreal, Canada